INTENSIVE CARE

INTENSIVE CARE

A THIN LINE BETWEEN SURVIVAL AND DEHUMANIZATION

Dr YOGESH MANHAS

Contributing Author: Dr. Abhijit Nair

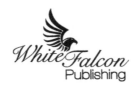

Intensive Care
Yogesh Manhas

Published by White Falcon Publishing

All rights reserved
First Edition, 2023
© Yogesh Manhas, 2023
Cover design by White Falcon Publishing, 2023
Cover image source freepik.com

No part of this publication may be reproduced, or stored in a retrieval system, or transmitted in any form by means of electronic, mechanical, photocopying or otherwise, without prior written permission from the publisher.

The contents of this book have been certified and timestamped on the Gnosis blockchain as a permanent proof of existence.
Scan the QR code or visit the URL given on the back cover to verify the blockchain certification for this book.

The views expressed in this work are solely those of the author and do not reflect the views of the publisher, and the publisher hereby disclaims any responsibility for them.

Requests for permission should be addressed to the publisher.

ISBN -978-1-63640-941-2

आरोग्यं परमं भाग्यं स्वास्थ्यं सर्वार्थसाधनम्॥

Being healthy is the ultimate destiny and with health,
all other works are accomplished.

*Dedicated to the patients and their families who place
trust in the ICU doctors and nurses.*

PREFACE

In the era of highly specialized organ-specific medical branches, there is a tendency to treat patients as diseased organs, forgetting that the diseased organ belongs to a human. A human who goes through varied emotions of fear, anger, anxiety, despondency, and uncertainty due to their illness. Moreover, evidence-based medicine, which is driven by large population sample statistics, tends to ignore the individuality of the patient. Intensive care is a highly complex and technologically advanced specialty that provides life support to critically ill patients. Since the Copenhagen polio epidemic, there has been rapid progress in the field of intensive care, and there is an ever-increasing demand for intensive care beds. The recent COVID-19 pandemic saw a huge rush of critically ill patients in need of intensive care beds.

Though intensive care saves lives, it is invasive and has the potential to cause harm. Patients in intensive care units are at risk of dehumanization as they lose control over their faculties. Families of patients go through immense psychological and emotional stress. In such scenarios, compassion and sensitivity of the intensive care team are needed to help mitigate the ordeal of the patients and their families.

This book is about acknowledging patients as humans, respecting their emotions, and maintaining their dignity while managing their illness. The book also intends to make the public aware of the various nuances of intensive care so that they can make informed decisions while availing themselves of intensive care services.

ACKNOWLEDGEMENT

First of all, I want to thank my parents who not only provided me with all the necessities but also imparted moral and ethical values. They live a simple and frugal life but ensured that their children got a good education and became independent.

I thank my wife, Dr. Tasvinder Kour, and son, Aryan Singh Manhas, for their unconditional support and love. They are my strength and greatest source of happiness.

I also thank my brothers and sisters who always stood by me.

I must acknowledge that the idea of writing a book was conceived by my colleague and dear friend, Dr. Abhijit Nair, who urged me to pen down my thoughts about intensive care. He has contributed to writing chapters of the book and helped me with his suggestions. I thank him for encouraging me to write.

I extend gratitude to my colleagues and intensive care team who are excellent co-workers. I learn new things from them each day and we are a proud team.

I hope the book serves its intended purpose.

TABLE OF CONTENTS

Chapter 1 Intensive care unit 1

Chapter 2 Intensivist... 4

Chapter 3 Critical care nurse 11

Chapter 4 Family of the Patient 16

Chapter 5 Dehumanization.. 20

Chapter 6 Humanizing intensive care 27

Chapter 7 Safety and quality of care............................. 35

Chapter 8 Rationalization of intensive care 53

Chapter 9 Do Not Resuscitate (DNR), Withholding and
Withdrawal of care. (End of life decisions)............... 62

Chapter 10 Peaceful transition from life to death 71

Chapter 11 Post-Intensive Care Rehabilitation 78

Chapter 12 Burnout among ICU staff 88

Chapter 13 Making Sense of Randomized controlled trials
in intensive care... 96

Chapter 14 Anecdotes 105

CHAPTER 1

INTENSIVE CARE UNIT

Dr Yogesh Manhas

The intensive care unit (ICU) is a specialized section of the hospital that has all the necessary monitoring and therapeutic equipment, as well as a team of skilled professionals who can manage critically ill patients requiring life support. Ideally, there is one trained nurse for each patient in the ICU, as well as round-the-clock intensivist doctors, respiratory therapists, physiotherapists, clinical pharmacists, and dieticians.

The concept of ICU can be traced back to Nurse Florence Nightingale, who observed during the Crimean War in 1850 that some soldiers required close and frequent monitoring. She created separate areas close to the nursing station for those who were severely injured which, apart from improving patient care, was a smart ergonomics that reduced the workload of nurses.[1]. A nurse who otherwise had to run around the ward could now observe seriously injured soldiers from the nursing station. In 1927, Dr. Walter Dandy, a neurosurgeon, created separate units for postoperative care of neurosurgical patients[2]. During the 2nd World War, shock units were created for injured soldiers. Until 1950, the concept of ICU was limited to a designated space with specialized nursing to take care of a particular group of patients. During the polio epidemic in 1952, separate units were created to ventilate paralyzed patients[3].

Patients with respiratory paralysis were ventilated in Drinker-Shaw "iron lungs" and with chest cuirasses. Due to a shortage of ventilators during the polio epidemic, paralyzed victims who had tracheostomy were manually ventilated. It required 200 medical students to manually ventilate patients round the clock for several weeks. Traditionally, it

2 Intensive Care

was anaesthesiologists who were tasked to manage patients requiring ventilator support because of their experience in ventilating patients in the operating room.

Since then, intensive care has evolved and become very complex with advancements in the knowledge of critical illness and increasing use of technology with modern monitors and life support equipment.

Acute severe illnesses such as septic shock, lung failure, heart failure, stroke, polytrauma, and others that were once fatal can now be survived with intensive care. While there is no doubt that intensive care saves lives, the mention of the ICU can create feelings of unease and intimidation among patients and their relatives. The current form of the intensive care unit can be a potentially hostile environment for patients and their relatives. Patients in the ICU are often connected to monitors by several leads that beep continuously in sync with the patient's vital parameters. Depending on the severity of the illness, the patient may be sedated and connectedS to a ventilator through a tube placed in their mouth. There is also a tube placed through the nose to feed and another tube that goes into the urinary bladder to measure hourly urine output. Additionally, there may be catheters in the neck or groin to infuse multiple drugs into the veins necessary to maintain the patient's vital functions.

Patients are socially isolated and restricted, and to make matters worse, they cannot communicate when connected to a ventilator. Thus, they are usually kept sedated, which further disorients them to time, place, and person. Once sedation is stopped, the patient may experience a variety of fears and anxieties. The absence of family, unfamiliar surroundings, uncertainty about life, inability to convey their thoughts, and loss of control over faculties are harrowing. The patient is completely dependent upon medical staff for their daily needs, such as hygiene, mouth care, turning in bed, feeding, etc.

Relatives also suffer from anxiety and helplessness due to restricted visiting hours to the ICU and their inability to participate in the care of their loved ones. Many ICUs mandate relatives to wear masks during visits, which makes it difficult for patients to recognize their loved ones who may be under the lingering effects of sedatives. Delirium, an acute and fluctuating disturbance of consciousness and cognition, has an incidence of up to 80% in ICU patients [4].

The book is an attempt to describe what intensive care is and what can be done to make it more meaningful and patient/family friendly.

REFERENCES:

1. KarimI H, MasoudiAlavI N. Florence Nightingale: The Mother of Nursing. Nurs Midwifery Stud. 2015; 4(2):e29475.
2. Firor WM. Walter E. Dandy: 1886-1946. Ann Surg. 1947; 126(1):113-5.
3. Ristagno G, Weil MH: History of critical care medicine: the past, present and future. In Intensive and Critical Care Medicine. Edited by Gullo A, Lumb PD, Besso J, Williams GF. Milan: Springer-Verlag; 2009:3-17.)
4. Ely WE, ShintanI A, Truman B et al. Delirium as a predictor of mortality in mechanically ventilated patients in the intensive care unit. J Am Med Assoc 2004; 291: 1753–62.

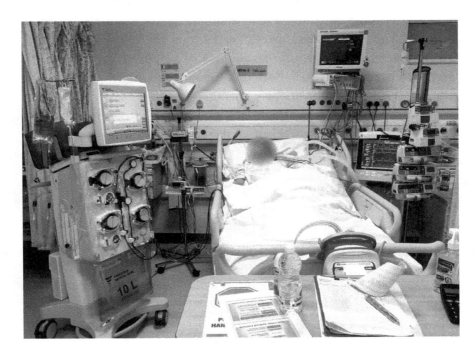

A patient in intensive care unit

CHAPTER 2

INTENSIVIST

Dr Yogesh Manhas

An Intensivist, also known as a critical care physician, is a specialist who manages critically ill patients admitted to an ICU. The ICU is usually a part of a multi-specialty hospital where there is access to laboratory, radiology, and blood bank services, along with various other medical specialties. Intensive care aims to promptly correct altered physiology due to illness so that further damage to organs can be halted while extensive investigative efforts are made to find the cause of an illness. This allows for a definitive treatment to be started. The various life-sustaining therapies used by Intensivists include mechanical ventilation to support the lungs, continuous hemodialysis to support the kidneys, and various medications given continuously through veins to support the heart and blood pressure. Sometimes, equipment like intra-aortic balloon pumps and ECMO (extracorporeal membrane oxygenation) are used to support heart and lung functions temporarily.

A patient in his mid-fifties presents to the Accident and Emergency Department with altered sensorium and difficult breathing. The intensivist receives a call to attend to him. Upon examination, the intensivist finds that the patient is unconscious and has low oxygenation levels and blood pressure. He immediately instructs that the patient needs to be intubated and put on a ventilator. Simultaneously, intensivist instructs to rush intravenous fluids and infuse medications to maintain the patient's blood pressure. Once the patient attains some stability, he is escorted to the intensive care unit. The intensivist assesses the patient again and decides upon the necessary investigations to find out the cause of the patient's critical condition. He also takes a history from family members and finds out that the patient had a fever for the past few days. So he decides to start empirical antibiotics. The patient's blood gas reveals severe hypoxia despite being on 100% oxygen through the ventilator. His chest X-ray shows bilateral infiltrates suggesting severe lung infection. The intensivist decides to put the patient in a prone position, which requires a minimum of 4 healthcare workers to execute the procedure. Before doing that, he decides to insert a central line into one of the neck veins of the patient to have reliable intravenous access to infuse several medications which patient would need. The nursing staff prepares and assists the intensivist in doing so. After this, the patient is placed in a prone position for the next 12 hours, and the intensivist instructs the assigned nurse to repeat blood gas regularly and inform him so that he can adjust ventilator settings. Next, he sits with the family members and explains the patient's condition, apprises them of the care plan, and answers any queries that they may have. It takes anywhere between 4-6 hours to stabilize a critically ill patient admitted to ICU. The next day, the intensivist is informed that the patient has not passed any urine since admission, and his renal function has significantly worsened. So he decides to start continuous renal replacement therapy (CRRT) as the patient cannot tolerate conventional hemodialysis due to a very low blood pressure. He then places a dialysis catheter into one of the large veins of the patient to initiate CRRT. This is one example of how an intensivist works and what kind of patients they deal with.

Critical illness can affect every organ of the body, including the brain, heart, kidneys, lungs, and liver. Therefore, intensivists require a comprehensive understanding of the interplay between various organs. They take a holistic approach rather than concentrating on specific organ functions. Intensivists also need to maintain a close communication and coordinate care with other specialties, seeking their opinions as necessary.

The role of an intensivist is to not only institute medical management but also ensure that the process of care within the ICU is well-organized to reduce the chances of human errors. Various teams, including intensivists, nurses, respiratory therapists, physiotherapists,

6   Intensive Care

and various experts from other specialties, work together to manage a critically ill patient. Coordinating them all requires good managerial abilities. Thus, intensivists must possess good administrative leadership in areas such as quality assurance, implementation of protocols, checklists, infection control policies, developing and auditing quality indicators, education, and research. ICUs need to work like a well-oiled machine to deliver quality care. The more organized an ICU is, the better the quality of care.

Across the world, there is an increasing demand for ICU beds, but unfortunately, trained intensive care physicians are scarce. Many ICU units in the world are understaffed. The recent pandemic has exposed the shortage of intensive care doctors and nurses.

Training and organization of ICU care are heterogeneous. Some countries, such as Australia, New Zealand, Switzerland, and Spain, recognize intensive care as the primary specialty, while in others, such as America and Europe, it is considered a subspecialty. India has recently introduced DM and DNB critical care courses as a super specialty. Primary specialty means that there is a specific curriculum and training program that can be accessed after completing graduation, usually lasting 5-6 years. Super and sub-specialty training programs can be entered upon completion of primary specialties such as Anaesthesiology, Medicine, Pulmonology, or Surgery. The primary specialty model has the benefit of a structured and focused training program, while super and sub-specialty programs are more flexible and bring the much-valued experience of different specialties into intensive care medicine.

Adding to the training heterogeneity is the structural variability. Some hospitals have mixed units wherein critically ill patients from various specialties are managed in a single ICU by a dedicated team while others have separate specialty ICU like medical, surgical, neurological, cardiac, obstetric, etc. managed by a team from the respective specialties. Though studies are reporting better outcomes with specialty units, particularly neuro-intensive care units, on a closer look, it may not be true. For example, one of the studies often quoted to argue for better care in neuro-intensive care units is by

Diringer and Edwards. However, there was a significant difference in the availability of a full-time intensivist in the intensive care units compared. Significantly more neuro units had the full-time intensivist as compared to general ICUs [1].

The separate specialty ICU is one of the most inefficient structural models for the following reasons. It results in duplication of infrastructure and manpower resources. ICU care remains heterogeneous which prevents the implementation of various policies necessary to improve the quality of care. Such an arrangement also affects intensive care training due to a lack of uniformity in care. Moreover, specialty ICU has not been shown to result in better outcomes in a large study [2]. Furthermore, whether a unit is closed or open also makes a difference in the quality of care delivered.

OPEN VERSUS CLOSED ICU MODEL. WHICH ONE IS BETTER?

ICU operates based on two organizational models: open, where the primary physician/surgeon decides to admit a patient to the ICU and is primarily responsible for the care, and where an intensivist provides consultation when asked for.

In the closed ICU model, patient care is primarily provided by Intensivists, with other specialties, including primary physicians, providing consultation when referred to them. The closed model requires a competent intensivist to be present continuously, 24 hours a day and 7 days a week. The closed ICU is led by trained and experienced intensivists.

There is enough evidence that closed ICUs provide better care with better outcomes [3].

The results of a recent systematic review and meta-analysis revealed that a closed ICU has lower death rates [4].

The vast majority of ICUs in the West are run in a closed format except for the USA.

8 Intensive Care

There is a lack of continuity in the open model as physicians/surgeons are committed to running outpatient clinics and looking after the ward patients. Since individual physicians/surgeons admit their patients in ICU in an open model, there is no central leadership. Moreover, though physicians/surgeons have expertise in their field, they do not have sufficient training as far as intensive care is concerned.

A closed ICU, on the other hand, provides continuity of care as there is a dedicated team of intensivists providing 24x7 coverage. This results in better coordination of services, a coherent treatment strategy, and efficient use of resources. Infection control policies are better implemented and audited in a closed ICU. Nurses feel less stressed and more confident in a closed ICU compared to an open ICU where they have to handle conflicting management plans between the primary physician and Intensivist. This has been reported in a study [5].

Despite good evidence in favor of closed ICUs improving patient outcomes, many hospitals are reluctant to implement the closed model. There are several reasons for it.

First, there is a lack of trained manpower. Despite the significant increase in the need for intensive care, formal training for doctors and nurses in this field began late and has not kept up with the rising demand.

Second, resistance comes from the physicians who see themselves as competent to manage critical patients, though they have limitations in handling critically ill patients which they fail to acknowledge. A closed ICU makes them feel redundant. There are financial concerns too, as physicians see it as the loss of their patients.

Private hospitals are also not in favor of a closed system because they need to hire a complete team of intensivists, both at junior and senior levels, to provide round-the-clock coverage, along with a nurse-to-patient ratio of 1:1. This necessitates significant investment and recurring costs, which prevent private players from adopting a closed model, despite evidence that it benefits patients.

Some experts have proposed a semi-closed ICU model in which Intensivists provide direct patient care in collaboration with physicians who are privileged to write orders. In this model, treating physicians remain actively involved in patient care. However, this model can be described as "too many cooks spoil the broth" as there are no clear duties and responsibilities outlined. At times, there is no clear leader, and everyone involved wants to take charge. Proponents of this model invoke the team concept, but the team can only function well when each member knows their responsibilities and limitations clearly.

REFERENCES:

1. Diringer MN, Edwards DF. Admission to a neurologic/neurosurgical intensive care unit is associated with a reduced mortality rate after intracerebral hemorrhage. Crit Care Med. 2001;29(3):635-40.

2. Nguyen YL, Milbrandt EB. Are specialized ICUs so special? Crit Care. 2009;13(5):314.

3. Pronovost PJ, Angus DC, Dorman T, Robinson KA, Dremsizov TT, Young TL. Physician staffing patterns and clinical outcomes in critically ill patients: a systematic review. JAMA. 2002; 288(17):2151-62.

4. Yang Q, Du JL, Shao F. Mortality rate and other clinical features observed in Open vs closed format intensive care units: A systematic review and meta-analysis. Medicine (Baltimore). 2019; 98(27):e16261.

5. Carson SS, Stocking C, PodsadeckI T, Christenson J, Pohlman A, MacRae S, Jordan J, Humphrey H, Siegler M, Hall J. Effects of organizational change in the medical intensive care unit of a teaching hospital: a comparison of 'open' and 'closed' formats. JAMA. 1996; 276(4):322-8.

10 Intensive Care

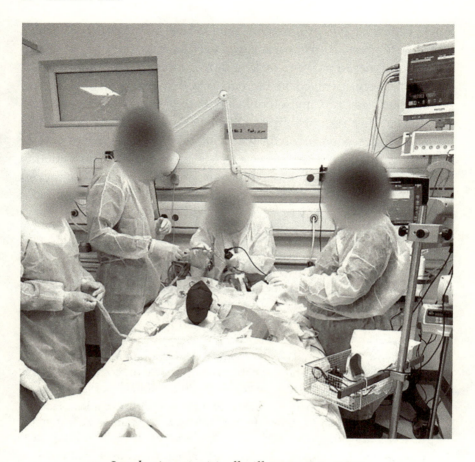

Intubating a critically ill patient in ICU

CHAPTER

3

CRITICAL CARE NURSE

Dr. Yogesh Manhas

Nurses in the ICU have one of the most difficult jobs. The care of critically ill patients is complex, and nursing responsibilities involve both physical and mental work that is exhaustive. Nurses are the backbone of Intensive care. The world acknowledges the contribution of Nurse Florence Nightingale to the concept of Intensive care. Apart from carrying out Intensivist orders, they are the first responders during acute deteriorations in patients' conditions when they make quick assessments and take decisions. ICU nurses assist intensivists with various procedures like central venous cannulation, bronchoscopy, endotracheal intubations, tracheostomy, cardioversion, etc. They manage complex life support equipment like ventilators, continuous renal replacement therapy (CRRT) machines, extracorporeal membrane oxygenators (ECMO), and intra-aortic balloon pumps (IABP). This requires detailed knowledge not only of the equipment but its complex interaction with patients' organs and the resulting homeostasis. Physical work includes cleaning and bathing patients, changing bed sheets, handling patients' body fluids/excreta, and turning patient positions every two hours. Many a times, nurses identify and timely correct errors committed by other professionals. Nurses interact closely with the patient and their families and form bonds with them. Thus, among caregivers, they are the most affected by the outcome of the patient.

Critical care nurses are also involved in caring for ward patients as team leaders of the critical care outreach team. They assess patients who are at risk of deterioration and assist ward nurses in managing them or transferring them to the ICU. Additionally, they follow up on

12   Intensive Care

patients who are moved from the ICU to step-down units or wards. Many nurses have taken on the roles of ICU managers, administrators, educators, and have also led clinical research with success.

Critical care nurses should possess a comprehensive knowledge base, be capable of addressing the intricate requirements of critically ill patients, possess the proficiency to make quick and sound clinical judgments, exhibit proficiency in both technological and compassionate aspects, and be equipped to handle ethical dilemmas. The World Health Organization (WHO) has developed a critical care nursing curriculum for WHO Europe [1].

The Indian Nursing Council has been offering a postgraduate diploma in critical care since 1993. Additionally, the Indian government has recently introduced a two-year course for critical care nurse practitioners[2].

On completion of the program, the Nurse Practitioner shall be able to:

1. Assume responsibility and accountability to provide competent care to critically ill patients and appropriate family care in tertiary care centers.
2. Demonstrate clinical competence and expertise in providing critical care, which includes diagnostic reasoning, complex monitoring, and therapies.
3. Apply theoretical, pathophysiological, and pharmacological principles and evidence base in implementing therapies/interventions in critical care
4. Identify the critical conditions and carry out interventions to stabilize and restore the patient's health and minimize or manage complications
5. Collaborate with other healthcare professionals in the critical care team, across the continuum of critical care.

Most of the ICUs in the world face a shortage of trained nurses. Due to the lack of adequately trained critical care nurses, many hospitals hire nurses who have just completed their basic nursing course and have no prior experience in ICU. Meanwhile, experienced or trained nurses prefer to move to high-income countries due to the significant income gap for critical care nurses compared to Western countries. This creates an imbalance in the quality of critical care worldwide. Additionally, nurses who are not trained in ICU care cannot handle a heavy workload and are prone to burnout, which increases the likelihood of fatal human errors.

The nurse-to-patient ratio is a crucial factor in determining the quality of care in the ICU. Due to the workload, ICUs require a one-to-one nurse-patient ratio, but unfortunately, few hospitals meet this requirement. To provide continuous 24-hour coverage, at least seven nurses are needed for each ICU bed. However, hospital managers often argue for a lower nurse-to-patient ratio, perhaps due to a lack of understanding of the ICU care process and the needs of critically ill patients. The number of required nursing staff is determined by several patient factors, such as the severity of illness, agitation, restlessness, body weight, frequency of observations, and the number of equipment supporting the patient. For instance, an obese patient on ventilator support who is agitated and combative may require more than one nurse to manage.

Not only are nurses required in adequate numbers, but they must also be qualified and experienced to deliver safe and effective intensive care. Several studies have documented that lower nurse staffing increases the risk of adverse events. One study found that a reduction in nurse staffing significantly increases the duration of weaning from mechanical ventilation [3]. Another study has shown that reduced ICU staffing results in increased postoperative pulmonary and infectious complications in patients with oesophageal resection [4]. Morrison and colleagues conducted a study to see the effects of nursing staff inexperience on the quality of care and outcomes. They found that nursing inexperience was responsible for 10% of all adverse incidents reported in a national database [5].

Though a 1:1 nurse-to-patient ratio is highly desirable in an ICU setting, it may not be cost-effective. This depends on the case mix and severity of the illness. Additionally, the experience of the nurse is

14 Intensive Care

a factor. A qualified, experienced nurse may be able to handle more than one critically ill patient compared to a less experienced nurse. There are scoring systems, such as the Therapeutic Intervention Scoring System (TISS) and Nine Equivalents of Nursing Manpower use score (NEMS), which can be used to fairly allocate nursing staff. [6,7]

ICU work is extremely difficult and exhausting. Moreover, ICU nurses are at great risk of occupational-related hazards, whether it be exposure to a variety of infectious agents, needle stick injuries, or physical trauma while moving beds, trolleys, or changing the position of patients who are sometimes morbidly obese. Shift work patterns not only take a toll on their health but also affect their personal and family life. Thus, nurses working in the ICU need a good working environment, decent monetary compensation, and reasonable working hours to balance their personal and professional life. Every effort must be made to prevent burnout among ICU nurses as it can adversely impact patient care.

REFERENCES:

1. https://apps.who.int/iris/handle/10665/107520
    WHO Europe critical care nursing curriculum: WHO European strategy for continuing education for nurses and midwives, 2003.
    (Last accessed on 1st March 2023)
2. https://main.mohfw.gov.in/sites/default/
    files/57996154451447054846_0.pdf
    Indian Nursing Council-Nurse practitioner in critical care (Post graduate- residency programme)
3. Thorens JB, Kaelin RM, Jolliet P, Chevrolet JC. Influence of the quality of nursing on the duration of weaning from mechanical ventilation in patients with chronic obstructive pulmonary disease. Crit Care Med. 1995;23(11):1807-15.
4. AmaravadI RK, Dimick JB, Pronovost PJ, Lipsett PA. ICU nurse-to-patient ratio is associated with complications and resource use after esophagectomy. Intensive Care Med. 2000;26(12):1857-62.
5. Morrison AL, Beckmann U, Durie M, Carless R, Gillies DM. The effects of nursing staff inexperience (NSI) on the occurrence of adverse patient experiences in ICUs. Aust Crit Care. 2001;14(3):116-21.

6. Cullen DJ, Civetta JM, Briggs BA, Ferrara LC. Therapeutic intervention scoring system: a method for quantitative comparison of patient care. Crit Care Med. 1974;2(2):57-60.
7. Reis Miranda D, Moreno R, Iapichino G. Nine equivalents of nursing manpower use score (NEMS). Intensive Care Med. 1997;23(7):760-5.

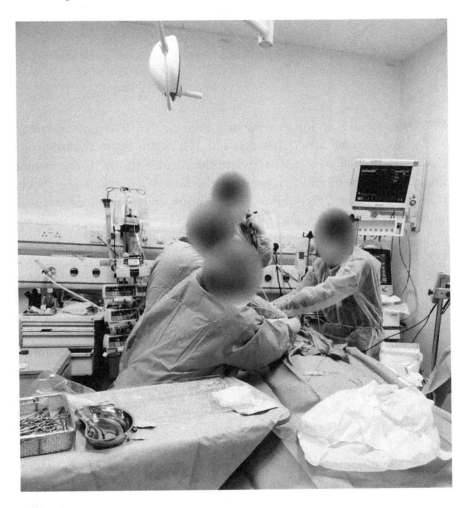

Performing percutaneous tracheostomy

CHAPTER 4

FAMILY OF THE PATIENT

Dr Yogesh Manhas

The family of the patient admitted to the ICU goes through an extreme level of stress. The ICU team must acknowledge and make efforts to alleviate the mental agony of the family. The various emotional reactions of the family described are shock, anxiety, confusion, irritability, anger, guilt, frustration, depression, numbness, uncertainty, and abandonment [1].

The personal lives of family members are disrupted when a loved one is admitted to the ICU. Patients in the ICU are often unable to communicate due to illness, hemodynamic instability, or sedative medications. As a result, the family is asked by the intensivists to make decisions on behalf of the patient. Additionally, ICU staff may approach the family to obtain consent for life support procedures. The uncertainty surrounding the patient's health can increase the anxiety and fear experienced by family members, making it difficult for them to make decisions. Studies have shown that family members often feel anxious, distressed, and helpless in these situations [2].

Family members may experience mental and physical exhaustion. It may affect their work, social interactions, and financial position. In one study, as many as 50% of informal caregivers either quit their job or reduce work hours. These collective effects on family members are known as Post Intensive Care Syndrome - Family (PICS-Family) [3].

A study reported that the prevalence of post-traumatic stress disorder among family members is up to 56.8% during ICU stay and up to

80% a year after discharge from ICU. Between 8-32% of close family members start using medications to control anxiety, depression, or insomnia after the ICU admission of their relative [4].

The above data emphasizes the importance of dealing with family members with sensitivity and compassion. A lack of empathy in the actions and language of ICU staff can heighten their anxiety and fears.

The Critical Care Family Needs Inventory (CCFNI), developed by Molter in 1979, is a tool for nurses to document the needs of family members in a critical care setting [5]. A Belgian study using the CCFNI tool has reported the needs of family members in order of their priority. The need for "information" was at the top [6], followed by "Assurance" and "Accessibility" to the patient. "Support" and "Comfort" were the least priority.

The two important needs of the family are being informed about the patient and assurance. It is the responsibility of the intensivist and ICU nursing staff to keep the family updated about the patient's condition. Information provided must be accurate and consistent among the ICU team. As far as assurance is concerned, it should be realistic and one must avoid giving false hopes. However, the family must be assured that everything possible will be done keeping the best interests of the patient. Moreover, assurance to protect the dignity and ensuring the comfort of the patient helps the family to cope better. This helps the ICU team to build a trusting relationship with the families of the patient which helps to avoid conflict in the goals of management. Families who lose trust in ICU staff have difficulty coping, are reluctant to ask questions, and are overall dissatisfied [7]. Compassion and good communication with family also help to avoid situations of violence and the use of abusive language against healthcare staff.

One of the worst things that can damage relations with the relatives of the patient is a contradictory statement about the patient's condition made by team members. It is an observation that this happens more often in an open ICU model though no studies have looked into this particular aspect. However, there is evidence to suggest that families are more satisfied concerning courtesy, compassion, and respect shown by the staff in a closed ICU [8].

Counseling a patient's relative is an important aspect of intensive care. The counseling room needs to be quiet, separate from the main area of the ICU, and have comfortable chairs/sofas, drinking water, and tissue boxes. Counseling in the doctor's room, bedside, or common area causes distractions, and relatives may feel inhibited to express themselves.

Listening to the family is important. They may provide information about the patient's medical history, beliefs, likes, dislikes, and idiosyncrasies that help to fine-tune the care of the patient. It also provides an opportunity to assess their expectations, apprehensions, and any psychological support that they may need.

Communication of ICU staff with the family, apart from providing information about the condition of their loved ones, must establish a positive relationship.

Accessibility of the patient's family in the ICU is restricted. Relatives are allowed twice a day to visit the patient. This is more a convention than of any scientific value. Rather there are studies to show that when relatives were involved in the provision of patient care, it resulted in more family satisfaction and less emotional distress [9,10].

REFERENCES:

1. Hughes F, Bryan K, Robbins I. Relatives' experiences of critical care. Nurs Crit Care. 2005; 10(1):23-30.
2. Paul F, Rattray J. Short- and long-term impact of critical illness on relatives: literature review. J Adv Nurs. 2008; 62:276-92.
3. Davidson JE, Jones C, Bienvenu OJ. Family response to critical illness: post-intensive care syndrome-family. Crit Care Med. 2012;40:618–24.
4. van Beusekom I, Bakhshi-Raiez F, de Keizer NF, Dongelmans DA, van der Schaaf M. Reported burden on informal caregivers of ICU survivors: a literature review. Crit Care. 2016; 20:16.

5. Molter NC. Needs of relatives of critically ill patients: a descriptive study. Heart Lung. 1979; 8(2):332-9.

6. Delva D, Vanoost S, Bijttebier P, Lauwers P, Wilmer A. Needs and feelings of anxiety of relatives of patients hospitalized in intensive care units: implications for social work. Soc Work Health Care. 2002;35(4):21-40.

7. Fry S, Warren NA. Perceived needs of critical care family members: a phenomenological discourse. Crit Care Nurs Q. 2007; 30(2):181-8.

8. Hwang DY, Yagoda D, Perrey HM, et al. Assessment of satisfaction with care among family members of survivors in a neuroscience intensive care unit. J NeurosciNurs. 2014; 46(2):106-16.

9. Mitchell M, Chaboyer W, Burmeister E, Foster M. Positive effects of a nursing intervention on family-centered care in adult critical care. American Journal of Critical Care. 2009; 18(6):543-52.

10. Appleyard ME, Gavaghan SR, Gonzalez C, Ananian L, Tyrell R, Carroll DL. Nurse-coached intervention for the families of patients in critical care units. Critical Care Nurse. 2000; 20(3):40-8.

CHAPTER 5

DEHUMANIZATION

Dr Yogesh Manhas

Dehumanization is the act of denying people their humanness. It is commonly associated with wars, conflicts, and racial discrimination, but little attention is paid to dehumanization in medical practice. Patients and their families are especially susceptible.

Humanness is defined by two characteristics: Uniquely Human and Human Nature.

Uniquely human traits are civility, refinement, morality, rationality, and maturity.

Human nature traits include emotional responsiveness, interpersonal warmth, cognitive openness, individuality, and depth.

Two types of dehumanization exist as described by Nick Haslam [1].

Animalistic dehumanization occurs when uniquely human traits are denied to an individual. People are seen as uncultured, backward, and unintelligent.

Mechanistic dehumanization occurs when human nature traits are denied to an individual. In this case, people are denied emotionality, warmth, cognitive openness, and individual agency. Here, people are perceived as objects, automaton machine-like.

Patients are vulnerable to dehumanization by healthcare staff, and they are subjected to a mechanistic form of dehumanization. The patients' individual beliefs and subjective experiences are neglected, and more reliance is given to the information provided by monitors and laboratory tests [2].

Patients are dehumanized by a lack of emotional touch and warmth, a quest for diagnosis of the disease while ignoring patients' subjective experience and when performing procedures on patients who have lost their autonomy.

The focus of medical education is to diagnose and treat illnesses, but there is very little attention paid to teach how to "care" for a patient. Evidence-based medicine, which tends to standardize care through the results of large sample statistics, also contributes to dehumanization to a certain extent by ignoring the individuality of patients.

The various reasons described for dehumanization in medical practice are:

1. De-individuation occurs when a patient becomes part of a group of patients and loses his/her individuality. Patients are dressed in the same type of gowns and are sometimes referred to by their bed number during handovers [3].
2. Perception of impaired patient agency due to illness. It makes healthcare staff assume that the patient is incapacitated and unable to make sound judgments, thus making them vulnerable to dehumanization.
3. Evidence-based medicine seeks the best evidence to guide the management of the patient, but it ignores the individuality and unique human characteristics of the patient.
4. Use of technology in medicine has numerous benefits but it also created a distance between doctor and patient. The use of monitors, remote relaying of the vital parameters, and availability of all laboratory and radiological results on personal computers make it less likely for the doctor to visit a patient at the bedside and interact with him.
5. Organ-specific specialization of medicine has changed the way a doctor perceives a patient. They tend to see the patient as diseased organs and focus only on their respective specialty. A holistic

22 Intensive Care

approach to the patient is lost in the era of specialization and super-specialization [4].

6. Lack of adequate infrastructure and manpower results in poor quality services, which is dehumanizing to the patients. Long waiting times, unhygienic and overcrowded clinics/hospitals cause distress among patients. Inadequate manpower overburdens the healthcare staff and creates an environment that dehumanizes not only patients but staff as well. Overburdened staff cannot exhibit empathy.

7. There are hospital rules and regulations that restrict family visits, prohibit home-cooked food, and do not allow children to visit hospitals.

8. Lack of empathy towards the patient

However, there is an interesting scientific aspect to reduced empathy among medical professionals. Neuroscientific studies have observed that indifference or being less empathetic can actually aid in complex clinical tasks.

YaweI Cheng et al conducted a study that found different areas of the brain were activated by acupuncture experts compared to non-experts when they were shown videos of needles being inserted into patients while their brain activity was mapped inside an MRI scanner. The study found that the areas of the brain associated with emotional processing of pain were less active in experts compared to non-experts, while areas of the brain involved in controlling emotions were more active in experts [5].

The human brain contains a Default Mode Network, which is also known as a Negative Task Network. This network is made up of various regions, including the medial parietal, posterior cingulate, medial prefrontal, lateral inferior parietal, and superior temporal cortices. In contrast to the Negative Task Network, there is also a Positive Task Network that includes areas in the dorsal parietal and lateral prefrontal cortices.These two networks function opposite to each other.

A study conducted by AI Jack et al demonstrated that tasks involving social reasoning and understanding the emotions and mental state of others activated the Negative Task Network and inhibited the Positive Task Network, whereas tasks involving physical cognition, such as reasoning about the mechanical properties of inanimate objects, activated the Positive Task Network and deactivated the Default Mode Network [6]. This could perhaps explain why there is reduced empathy among healthcare professionals towards patients while performing complex clinical interventions.

In clinical scenarios, it has been observed that an emotional response to a crisis can prevent effective management. For instance, when a patient experiences cardiac arrest, the team leader must focus on the steps of resuscitation and supervise team members to ensure timely and effective resuscitation, which offers the best chance of the patient's survival. Similarly, when dealing with a bleeding patient, the surgeon's priority is to control the bleeding. Emotional responses in such situations can hinder performance. Therefore, mechanistic dehumanization, or the objectification of the patient, is possible when dealing with complex clinical problems.

In another study conducted by Capoza et al, it was found that oncology physicians and nurses assign a lower human status (animalistic dehumanization) to patients compared to themselves by ignoring the uniquely human characteristics of the patient [7].

Studies have postulated that this kind of dehumanization by healthcare staff is a coping mechanism for increased workplace stress [8].

Several other studies have linked dehumanization by medical professionals with their coping strategy for stress [9,10].

However, dehumanizing patients is a terrible coping mechanism. It not only adversely affects patients' well-being but also patient healthcare-provider relations. The negative consequences of implicit or explicit dehumanization of patients can induce a feeling of inferiority, guilt, and shame among patients. Patients feel angry, frustrated, and sad. It result in failure in compliance with their medications and follow-up as patients feel that their existence is not important [11].

DEHUMANIZING NATURE OF ICU CARE

The ICU environment can be dehumanizing for patients and their families. Patients admitted to the ICU are typically very ill and require life support measures. Upon admission, nurses and doctors quickly assess the patient's vital signs for any necessary resuscitative measures. Patients are often only greeted with a brief hello and informed that they are in the ICU. Family members are usually not allowed, and patients are surrounded by unfamiliar faces wearing masks. Due to their illness, patients may not be able to comprehend their surroundings. Nurses change patients into ICU gowns and connect them to monitors to measure blood pressure, heart rate, and oxygen saturation. Doctors may place a cannula into an artery to continuously monitor blood pressure. Cannulas are also placed into veins to administer fluids and medications. In some cases, a three or four-lumen catheter is placed into the jugular vein.

Patients who are unable to breathe and have low oxygen in their blood, or those in a coma, are supported by a ventilator. They are put to sleep, and an endotracheal tube is inserted into their trachea, which is then connected to the ventilator. Sometimes, intensivists prescribe paralyzing agents to facilitate mechanical ventilation. Imagine a situation where someone is paralyzed but can see, hear, and feel while being provided artificial breaths to stay alive. It is like a torture, and can happen in the ICU if patients who are paralyzed are not adequately sedated. A tube is placed into the stomach through the nose for feeding, and another is inserted into the bladder to monitor hourly urine output. Some patients require additional life support in the form of dialysis, Extracorporeal membrane oxygenation (ECMO), intra-aortic balloon pump (IABP), or a temporary pacemaker, depending on their clinical condition.

All of the life support interventions mentioned above are uncomfortable and cause distress and pain to the patient. Although patients are sedated and given powerful analgesics to minimize the unpleasantness of the ICU interventions, it cannot be completely eliminated. Sedatives and analgesics aim to keep the patient calm and cooperative, but in practice, this is seldom achieved. Either the patient is deeply sedated or becomes very restless and agitated when attempting to reduce sedation. Daily stopping or reduction of sedation to assess the patient's response is an evidence-based practice that helps prevent several complications, but every time sedation is stopped, the patient experiences discomfort and unpleasantness. At times, patients become so agitated that they need to be restrained.

Confined to the bed, patients in the ICU lose control of their bodies. They are completely dependent on ICU staff. It's difficult for them to communicate and convey what they want. Their bodies are exposed to the fixed temperature of the ICU. There is a sense of loss of dignity and privacy.

REFERENCES:

1. Haslam N. Dehumanization: an integrative review. Pers Soc Psychol Rev. 2006;10(3):252-64.
2. Lekka D, Richardson C, Madoglou A, et al. Dehumanization of Hospitalized Patients and Self-Dehumanization by Health Professionals and the General Population in Greece. Cureus. 2021; 13(12):e20182.
3. K Jenni, G Loewenstein. Explaining the Identifiable Victim Effect. Journal of Risk and Uncertainty. 1997; 235–257.
4. PawlikowskI M. Dehumanization of contemporary medicine: causes and remedies. Neuro Endocrinol Lett. 2002; 23(1):5-7; discussion 4.
5. Cheng Y, Lin CP, et al. Expertise modulates the perception of pain in others. Curr Biol. 2007; 17(19):1708-13.
6. Jack AI, Dawson AJ, Begany KL, et al. fMRI reveals reciprocal inhibition between social and physical cognitive domains. Neuroimage. 2013; 66:385-401.
7. Capozza D, Visintin EP, Falvo R, TestonI I. Dehumanization of the cancer patient in medical contexts. Salute e Società. 2015 Jan 1.
8. TrifilettI E, DI Bernardo GA, Falvo R, Capozza D. Patients are not fully human: A nurse's coping response to stress. Journal of Applied Social Psychology. 2014; 44(12):768-77.
9. Vaes J, Muratore M. Defensive dehumanization in the medical practice: a cross-sectional study from a health care worker's perspective. Br J Soc Psychol. 2013; 52(1):180-90.

10. Falvo R, ColledanI D, Capozza D. Denying full humanity to patients and nurses's wellL-being: The moderating role of attachment secuirty. TPM: Testing, Psychometrics, Methodology in Applied Psychology. 2021; 28(2021).

11. Bastian B, Haslam N. Experiencing dehumanization: Cognitive and emotional effects of everyday dehumanization. Basic and Applied Social Psychology. 2011; 33(4):295-303.

CHAPTER 6

HUMANIZING INTENSIVE CARE

Dr Yogesh Manhas

There is a compelling need to change the way intensive care is provided to make it more humane. It requires both structural and organizational changes. In this section, I shall discuss the required changes under three parts that can make ICU care more humanized.

INFRASTRUCTURE:

Perhaps the most important change required is in the design of intensive care units. The recommended space area for an ICU bed is 25 square meters, but very few intensive care units meet this requirement. Some units do not even have half the recommended area, and many units do not have any windows for natural light. Worse still are the isolation rooms that resemble solitary prisons. Considering the number of equipment that may be attached to patients for life support, the ICU area needs to be even bigger than the current recommendations. Overcrowded units are not only uncomfortable for patients and staff, but also increase the chances of the spread of hospital-acquired infections. The bed area should include space for at least one family member to be present, who can sit or lie comfortably on a couch. Each bed space must be separated from the next by a fixed soundproof partition to ensure privacy. The area in the patient's line of vision should be designed in a way that allows for the hanging of a clock, calendar, patient's family photographs, or pleasant murals. The provision of natural light through windows at each bed area helps maintain the circadian rhythm of both patients and ICU staff.

MANPOWER:

Adequate manpower is the most fundamental requirement for delivering quality care. It is not only important to have enough staff, but the staff working in the ICU must also be adequately trained and experienced in providing ICU care. Inadequate manpower can lead to the dehumanization of ICU staff, which in turn can lead to the dehumanization of patients. Overworked and overburdened staff are unable to provide compassionate care and be empathetic to patients. The staff themselves suffer from burnout, and their work becomes mechanized with less focus on the human aspect of care. Overworked staff prioritize their work in a way that essential tasks for patients are completed, while communication with patients, exploring their concerns and needs, and patient comfort take a backseat as these aspects of care are time-consuming. Additionally, overburdened staff are reluctant to reduce sedatives as an awake patient is more demanding. Improved working conditions for ICU staff can result in a more humane approach towards patients.

PROCESS OF CARE:

Changes in the way ICU care is delivered to the patient can help prevent dehumanization.

Approaching and greeting a patient with their name while examining during rounds is a gesture of humanization. Even if the patient is under sedation or comatose, it is courteous to greet and address them by their name. Addressing patients as room or bed numbers is very dehumanizing. Their dignity and privacy must be protected while examining, as there is a tendency to ignore while they are under sedation or in a coma.

Simple gestures like holding hands and assuring them may help prevent negative feelings in the patient.

The patient's needs should be attended to promptly. For example, if the patient has soiled himself, it must be cleaned immediately.

Staff should communicate with the patient and inform them of their location and reason for being there in order to orient them to time, place, and person. Patients who are recovering and no longer sedated may become more oriented and less agitated if they are given their glasses, hearing aids, and other necessary items.

Music and television in the patient area help create a friendly and acceptable environment.

Empathy is defined as the ability to understand others' emotions and feelings. It differs from sympathy, which involves sharing others' emotions. Empathy is not an inborn personality trait but can be taught and should be taught to medical students [1].

Competence among doctors and nurses is defined by the knowledge and skills that they possess, but the ability to care and empathize with patients should also be a part of the competence checklist during their training period.

Dr. Helen Reiss, an Associate Professor of Psychiatry at Harvard Medical School and Director of the Empathy and Relational Science Program at Massachusetts General Hospital, has conducted extensive research on the neurobiology of empathy. She founded Empathetics, an online course that teaches and develops empathy in physicians. There is good reason to instill empathy in medical professionals, as studies have shown that empathetic care leads to improved patient satisfaction, better adherence to treatment, improved clinical outcomes, enhanced mutual trust, and fewer legal suits against medical professionals [2-6].

In ICU settings, empathy is necessary not only for patients but also for their families who are experiencing high levels of stress and anxiety. However, the ICU is a complex environment where Intensivists must perform life-saving procedures that are often complicated. As previously discussed, when performing complex tasks, one may be less empathetic in order to focus on the task at hand. Therefore, intensivists may need to switch between being empathetic or less empathetic depending on the task they are performing.

30   Intensive Care

Communicating with the patient is particularly challenging in the ICU. Patients who are ventilated cannot speak due to the tube in their trachea. Some patients may be able to write, but many cannot due to motor weakness or the lingering effects of sedatives. Neurological disorders and head and neck trauma impair the ability to speak and write. It is frustrating for the patient, family, and ICU staff. Imagine a patient who is critically ill and likely to die, unable to communicate their last wishes and message to loved ones.

Most nurse-patient communication lasts less than one minute and is usually task-related information, a command, or a question [7]. The patient may try to communicate through gestures if they can move their hands or by facial expressions like grimacing when they are in pain. Sometimes they try mouthing words. Picture boards that depict the common needs of the patient are used when the patient can respond with yes or no by nodding their head or blinking their eyes. But all these methods are time-consuming and need commitment from the staff to actively engage themselves in communicating with the patients. Scientists are working on artificial intelligence technology that can synthesize speech by mapping the thoughts of the patient. If successful, it would bring a major change in ICU care [8].

Another distressing problem in the ICU is the noise that prevents patients from sleeping. The noise comes from a variety of sources, such as staff conversations, the noise of ventilators and dialysis machines, alarms from monitors, and various other equipment. The World Health Organization (WHO) recommends noise levels of 40 decibels in hospital settings. However, ICU noise levels can exceed 60 decibels [9,10].

ICU should have a strategy to lower noise levels, especially during nighttime. Lowering the volume or switching off unnecessary or low-priority alarms and the use of earplugs in patients can help prevent adverse effects of high levels of noise in intensive care units. Future technology may devise a system where the caring nurse can be alerted without having a noisy alarm system.

One of the dehumanizing features of intensive care units is restricted visiting times for the relatives and not allowing them to stay at the patient's bedside. Such policies have little scientific basis.

Don't we all want our loved ones to be by our side when we become ill? There is strong evidence from multiple observational studies that allowing families to visit freely during hospital hours enhances their satisfaction and contributes to the well-being of patients [11,12].

A randomized trial found that liberal visiting hours reduced cardiovascular complications and lowered anxiety among ICU patients [13].

Many hospitals have changed their visiting policies in an attempt to provide family and patient-centered ICU care. However, despite the potential benefits of a liberal visit policy, the majority of hospitals in the world still continue with restricted policies.

The following arguments are put forth by ICU staff for not implementing the liberal visitation policy:

Interference with the provision of care. However, studies have found that liberal visiting hours did not interfere with patient care significantly [14].

On the contrary, the presence of a family member observing the care provider may result in more conscientious care being provided. although this aspect has not yet been studied. Humans modify their behavior in response to their awareness of being observed which is known as Hawthorne effect.

Family members can be involved in the patient care process. They provide emotional support and assurance, and help in communicating with the patient. They can provide important medical history or personal likes and dislikes of the patient, which can help individualize the care. Family members can also help physically during bathing, changing positions, and massaging the patient. This provides intimacy to the patient and a feeling of warmth. It also provides an opportunity for the family to contribute to the patient's care, which may help them to overcome grief in case the patient succumbs to the illness [15].

The second argument is that a liberal visiting policy can increase the infection rate among ICU patients. Again, there is no real evidence for

32   Intensive Care

this. Rather, studies have shown that there is no increase in infection rate when liberal visits were allowed [13].

In an observational study, researchers attempted to determine if bacteria colonizing on family members were the cause of infections in patients. Swabs were taken from the noses and hands of family members, but no correlation was found between colonizing organisms on family members and the organisms causing infections in patients. It should be noted that all family members were instructed to wash their hands before and after visiting the patient.

Family members, if instructed properly and made aware of the potential for resistant infections that patients can acquire, perhaps they would be as careful in adhering to hand hygiene as ICU staff [16].

Another reason cited against liberal visits by family is the notion that family members may experience distress and stress being present during procedures and resuscitation, but studies have shown otherwise. A study found that an unrestricted visiting policy has a positive impact on 88% of families and reduces anxiety in 66% [17]. It also allows family members to adjust to their working schedule and other commitments.

In an interesting study conducted in France and published in The New England Journal of Medicine, patients' relatives were allowed to be present during cardiopulmonary resuscitation (CPR) [18]. The result showed that the incidence of post-traumatic stress disorder was less in those family members who witnessed the resuscitative efforts and their presence did not affect the performance of the medical team and did not result in any medico-legal claims.

The evidence suggests that a liberal and open visiting policy benefits both patients and family members and reflects a humane approach on the part of the hospital organization. Moreover, apart from building trust between hospital staff and society, such a policy shall make people more aware of the work done in the ICU. I am sure that this will generate more respect and appreciation for the ICU staff.

Indeed, there are barriers to the implementation of liberal visiting policies but they can be addressed by structural and organizational changes. Often, resistance comes from doctors and nurses who are unwilling to accept a new concept. I recall an incident during an infection control meeting in a tertiary hospital when a surgeon criticized the inability of the ICU team to contain family visits and linked it to an increase in ICU-acquired infections. I argued that the presence of family can benefit the patient and family members can be educated about infection control and hand hygiene. Everyone in the meeting reacted as if I made an outrageous comment.

A study found that the barriers to liberal visiting time are lack of adequate patient bed space and the presence of relatives obstructing access to patients, lack of privacy and confidentiality, disruption of work rounds, and sometimes physical and emotional assault from difficult relatives. As discussed earlier, changes in the design of the ICU, education of family members through information leaflets containing rules and policies, and availability of security and social support are a few changes that can overcome barriers to liberal visiting policy [19].

REFERENCES:

1. Riess H, Kelley JM, Bailey RW, Dunn EJ, Phillips M. Empathy training for resident physicians: a randomized controlled trial of a neuroscience-informed curriculum. Journal of general internal medicine. 2012; 27(10):1280-6.
2. Hojat M, Louis DZ, Markham FW, Wender R, Rabinowitz C, Gonnella JS. Physicians' empathy and clinical outcomes for diabetic patients. Academic Medicine. 2011; 86(3):359-64.
3. Kim SS, Kaplowitz S, Johnston MV. The effects of physician empathy on patient satisfaction and compliance. Evaluation & the health professions. 2004; 27(3):237-51.
4. DiMatteo MR, Sherbourne CD, Hays RD, et al. Physicians' characteristics influence patients' adherence to medical treatment: Results from the medical outcomes study. Health Psych. 1993; 12:93–102.
5. Neuwirth ZE. Physician empathy—Should we care? Lancet. 1997; 350:606.
6. Squier RW. A model of empathetic understanding and adherence to treatment regimens in a practitioner–patient relationships. Soc Scl Med. 1990;30:325–339.

34 Intensive Care

7. Ashworth P, Carroll SM, Happ MB, Nelson J. Original SPEACS–Basic Communication Training Program References Communication problems in ICU and Assessment. Nursing Research. 2004;26:85-103.

8. AnumanchipallI GK, Chartier J, Chang EF. Speech synthesis from neural decoding of spoken sentences. Nature. 2019; 568(7753):493-8.

9. Simons KS, Verweij E, Lemmens P, et al. Noise in the intensive care unit and its influence on sleep quality: a multicenter observational study in Dutch intensive care units. Critical Care. 2018; 22(1):1-8.

10. Weinhouse GL, Schwab RJ, Watson PL, Patil N, Vaccaro B, Pandharipande P, Ely EW. Bench-to-bedside review: delirium in ICU patients-importance of sleep deprivation. Critical care. 2009; 13:1-8.

11. Berwick DM, Kotagal. Restricted visiting hours in ICUs. JAMA. 2004;292(6):736-737

12. Roland P, Russell J, Richards KC, Sullivan SC. Visitation in critical care: process and outcomes of a performance improvement initiative. J Nurs Care Qual. 2001;15(2):18-26.

13. FumagallI S, BoncinellI L, Lo Nostro A, et al. Reduced cardiocirculatory complications with unrestrictive visiting policy in an intensive care unit: results from a pilot, randomized trial. Circulation. 2006; 113(7):946-52.

14. Garrouste-Orgeas M, Philippart F, Timsit J, et al. Perceptions of a 24-hour visiting policy in the intensive care unit. Crit Care Med. 2008;36(1):30-35.

15. McAdam JL, AraI S, Puntillo KA. Unrecognized contributions of families in the intensive care unit. Intensive care medicine. 2008; 34:1097-101.

16. Malacarne P, PinI S, De Feo N. Relationship between pathogenic and colonizing microorganisms detected in intensive care unit patients and in their family members and visitors. Infection Control & Hospital Epidemiology. 2008; 29(7):679-81.

17. Simon SK, Phillips K, BadalamentI S, Ohlert J, Krumberger J. Current practices regarding visitation policies in critical care units. Am J Crit Care. 1997;6: 210-217.

18. Jabre P, Belpomme V, Azoulay E, Jacob L, Bertrand L, Lapostolle F, Tazarourte K, Bouilleau G, Pinaud V, Broche C, Normand D. Family presence during cardiopulmonary resuscitation. N Engl J Med. 2013; 368:1008-18.

19. Lee MD, Friedenberg AS, Mukpo DH, Conray K, Palmisciano A, Levy MM. Visiting hours policies in New England intensive care units: strategies for improvement. Critical care medicine. 2007; 35(2):497-501.

CHAPTER 7

SAFETY AND QUALITY OF CARE

Dr Yogesh Manhas

Quality is not easy to define and it is also not easy to provide. Quality is defined in various ways with regards to products, services, value, and both internal and external consumers.

"Primum non nocere," a Latin phrase meaning "first do no harm," is often quoted in the medical profession to emphasize the importance of safety in providing care to patients. However, intensive care unit is a place where almost every intervention has the potential to cause harm given the complex and complicated nature of intensive care. The Institute of Medicine is an American non-profit, non-governmental organization that provides evidence-based information and advice regarding health sciences to policymakers, professionals, and the public. On November 29, 1999, its publication titled "To Err is Human: Building a Safer Health System" reported that between 44,000 to 98,000 patients die every year in the United States of America as a result of medical errors. This report set in motion discussions about patient safety, identifying factors responsible and what can be done to mitigate errors.

The risk of errors is significantly greater in Intensive Care Units due to the high and variable workload, complex interaction between staff, patients, and equipment, complicated procedures, and shift work patterns involving handovers. Intensive care requires hundreds of steps to be performed accurately on a daily basis to achieve the desired outcome. A study published in 1995 discovered that ICU staff performs as many as 178 activities per patient per day, which explains the high workload and increased risk of human errors [1].

The Institute of Medicine, in its report "To Err is Human," defined error as either a failure of a planned action to be completed as intended or a wrong plan to achieve the aim [2].

The Safety Improvement for Patients in Europe Project (SIMPATIE Project) developed a European vocabulary that defines 24 terms related to patient safety. Some of the important definitions include:

Adverse event: An unintended and undesired occurrence in the healthcare process because of the performance or lack thereof of the healthcare provider and/or the healthcare system.

Actual Event: An adverse event that causes harm.

Near Miss: An adverse event with the capacity to cause harm but which does not have adverse consequences because of, for instance, timely and appropriate identification and correction of potential consequences for the patient. Near misses are important to recognize because they allow us to analyze and make corrections before near misses turn into actual events.

Sentinel event: Sentinel reflects the seriousness of the injury and the likelihood that investigation of an event will reveal a serious problem in current policies or procedures. Such events signal the need for immediate investigation and response.

Complication: An unintended and undesirable outcome that develops as a consequence of the intervention of an already present illness. It may be non-preventable under the given circumstances.

Critical incident: Occurrences that are significant or pivotal in either a desirable or undesirable way. Significant or pivotal means that there was significant potential for harm, but also that the event has the potential to reveal important hazards in the organization [3].

An observational, 24-hour cross-sectional study, including 205 intensive care units worldwide, found 584 medical errors affecting 391 patients out of a total of 1913 adult patients. The errors were medication-related, inadvertent dislodgement of catheters and drains, blockage of airway tubes, and equipment failure [4].

A study was conducted at a tertiary teaching hospital in Jerusalem to record error reports and activity profiles of nurses and physicians in ICU patients over a 4-month period. The study found a total of 554 human errors, of which 147 (29%) could potentially cause significant deterioration in the patient's status or even death. 46% of errors were committed by physicians and 54% by nursing staff. The study also found that more errors occurred during the daytime than at night, and peak errors coincided with peak activity of physicians and nurses. However, peaks also occurred during nurse shift changes [5].

A prospective observational study was conducted over one year in an eleven-bed multispecialty ICU, which recorded a total of 777 critical incidents [6]. Of the total incidents, 241 (31%) were due to human errors. Interestingly, all incidents that led to serious consequences were due to planning errors, which were defined as the use of a wrong plan to achieve an aim.

The above studies reflect the scale of the problem concerning the safety of patient care.

The Institute of Medicine has defined safety as the absence of clinical errors, either by commission or omission.

Safety improvement for patients in Europe (SIMPATIE) defines safety in terms of how to achieve it:

The continuous identification, analysis, and management of patient-related risks and incidents to make patient care safer and minimize harm to the patients. Safety emerges from the interaction of the components of the systems. Improving safety depends on learning how safety emerges from such interactions.

Quality and safety of care are often used interchangeably. The foremost goal of quality is indeed the safety of the patient, but quality has several other dimensions. The Institute of Medicine defined healthcare quality as "the degree to which health services for individuals and populations increase the likelihood of desired health outcomes and are consistent with current professional knowledge." The attributes of quality healthcare are safety, effectiveness, equity, timeliness, efficiency, and patient-centeredness.

All stakeholders, including the public, must understand what it takes to provide quality healthcare. The performance or competence of healthcare professionals alone does not determine the quality of healthcare. There are other equally important factors to consider. Often, there is a gap between expectations and understanding of the resources and efforts needed for quality healthcare.

Donabedian proposed a model to assess quality in three domains: Structure, Process, and Outcome [7].

The National Quality Measures Clearinghouse (NMQC) added two additional domains:

1. Experience of Care, which emphasizes the significance of patient perceptions.
2. Access to care that highlights the importance of timing in the provision of healthcare.

Let us discuss the importance of each domain:

Structure: Structure includes the design of the ICU, various equipment, and human resources. The importance of ICU design was discussed in the previous chapters. Lack of adequate space not only adversely affects infection control measures but also creates a negative work environment for the staff. Lack of natural light may increase the incidence of delirium among patients. There are studies to show the positive effect of natural light in preventing delirium among patients admitted to the ICU.

A retrospective study conducted in a university-affiliated hospital in Seoul found that the incidence of delirium was much lower among patients who were admitted to isolation rooms with a window than those who were in windowless rooms [8].

Another study in a French university hospital found that patients admitted to rooms with the provision of natural light through windows had less agitation and a reduced risk of hallucinations [9].

Hospital-acquired multidrug-resistant infections cause significant morbidity and mortality, as well as a huge financial burden due to the infections. The importance of ICU design is not appreciated enough, as structural design is not often mentioned in the literature as a factor in infection control in the ICU. A design that makes it difficult for hospital staff to carry infections from one patient to another should be given a thought. For example, a study showed that when the ICU was moved to a new facility with a single-room ICU design, there was a marked decrease in hospital-acquired infections with multidrug-resistant organisms compared to the open-bay ICU design [10].

Additionally, ICU should be designed in a way to maximize the convenience of the working staff. For example, there is a greater chance of hand hygiene compliance if the wash basin is located at each patient's bedside than if it is located at a distant place.

As far as design is concerned, it wouldn't be wrong to describe the majority of intensive care units as an ergonomic catastrophe. Very little attention is paid to human-machine interaction, a branch of science called Human Factor Engineering or Ergonomics. The ICU is a place where staff works with complicated machines to provide life support to critically ill patients, and thus there is a huge scope for human factor engineers to improve things to make the work environment safe for both care providers and patients [11].

40 Intensive Care

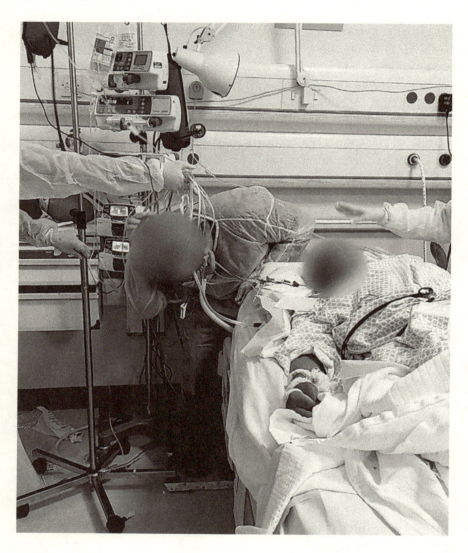

Numerous cables and infusion tubings are obstructing access to the head end of the patient.

I remember an incident when one of my colleagues was cannulating the internal jugular vein of a patient to place a central venous line. The patient was in an isolation room, which was small and had limited access. My colleague had to negotiate himself with great difficulty around numerous cables coming out of the wall sockets to reach the head end. The procedure turned out to be even more challenging, and he had to stand in that confined space for a bit longer. When I went inside to help him with the procedure, I suddenly found him sweating, and within seconds he collapsed onto the patient while holding the needle in his hand. Luckily, it did not hit him. The space was so narrow, with cables all around, that I could not get him off the patient, nor could I pull him out. Only after removing all the cables from the wall sockets could we pull him out and lay him flat with his legs up when he regained consciousness. This incident is an example of how the poor ergonomic design of the ICU can compromise the safety of healthcare staff and patients.

Inadequate human resources are a significant limiting factor for the safety and quality of care. A high workload and an increased number of complex interventions increase the chances of errors. Fatigue and sleep deprivation due to extended working hours, shift duties to provide 24x7 coverage, and inadequate duty off days to recover affect performance at work, particularly in those involving the use of higher cognitive abilities to make decisions. In a study, 56% of night shift nurses were sleep deprived. Moreover, in the same study, it was interesting to note that both sleep-deprived and non-sleep-deprived nurses had poor psychomotor performances when doing night shift duty. Working during night shifts alters diurnal patterns, which may have adverse effects on psychomotor performance [12].

A study conducted in New Zealand assessed fatigue-related risk among junior doctors who worked more than 40 hours a week. The study found that 24% of the doctors reported falling asleep while driving home, 66% had felt close to falling asleep at the wheel, and 42% recalled a fatigue-related clinical error in the past 6 months. The study also found that night work was independently associated with more fatigue [13].

In any profession where tolerance for errors is low and consequences of error are grave, the issue of fatigue is of major importance. Intensive care is one such field of medicine.

Nurses and physicians who worked 12-hour night shifts in the emergency department took part in a randomized controlled trial.

42   Intensive Care

One group was permitted to take a 40-minute nap at 3 AM. The study discovered that the group who took a nap had better performance and alertness at the end of their night shift compared to those who did not nap [14].

The above studies underline the importance of understanding human limits and emphasize that in order to provide safe and quality care, employer and hospital authorities must recruit enough staff to keep work hours reasonable with sufficient off-duty days for the night shift staff to ensure their optimal performance at work.

Unfortunately, the well-being of staff is often ignored in reality. For instance, at a private university hospital, the chairman objected to my request for a room to rest for the in-house resident doctor. He questioned why a doctor would need to rest while on duty. Additionally, he was displeased with residents receiving 24 hours off after working 16 hours, including night hours. This mindset of the authorities not only demonstrates ignorance but also a dehumanizing attitude towards doctors and nurses.

Process of care: The process of care refers to how ICU care is organized and delivered. It is the responsibility of the ICU team, led by the director of the ICU. The better the ICU is organized, the better the outcomes. The importance of an Intensivist-led closed ICU has already been discussed. An effective process of care is evidence-based and delivered appropriately and in a timely manner. Bundles of care, checklists, and protocols are used in the ICU to improve the process of care. This not only prevents morbidity and mortality but also reduces the cost of treatment.

For example, the implementation of ventilator weaning protocols by multidisciplinary teams was shown to save $13,132 per patient stay [15].

A bundle of care is a set of evidence-based interventions that, when delivered together, result in better outcomes than performing interventions individually. Surviving sepsis is an example of a bundle that includes measuring lactate levels in the blood, administering fluids, antibiotics, obtaining blood cultures, and using vasopressors within the first hour of a patient presenting with septic shock. Another example of a care bundle that improves outcomes is the prevention of ventilator-associated pneumonia. Ventilator-associated pneumonia is a lung infection that occurs in patients who are on mechanical ventilators for more than 48 hours. It causes significant morbidity and mortality and increases the cost of healthcare [16].

A study conducted in a Scottish ICU showed that there was a significant reduction in the incidence of ventilator-associated pneumonia after the implementation of preventive care bundles [17].

Protocols are predetermined steps of management that are specific to a disease, procedure, or event. Examples of protocols include the management of diabetic ketoacidosis, the ARDS network protocol for initiating ventilation in ARDS patients, replacement of potassium in Hypokalemia, and management of hyperkalaemia. Procedure-specific protocols include tracheostomy, bronchoscopy, and others. Studies have shown that implementing protocols in ICU care can lead to improved outcomes [18,19].

Despite the evidence, many clinicians are reluctant to accept the importance of protocols. They argue that protocols prevent the use of clinical judgment and make staff more complacent. However, I strongly disagree. Protocols ensure that a minimum basic standard of care is provided for a particular clinical condition or while doing a procedure. Given that any ICU has a staff of varying knowledge and clinical experience, having a protocol reduces the variability in management which is very important to ensure safety and quality of care. Moreover, it provides an opportunity for everyone to learn. Protocols make less experienced staff feel more confident in managing patients.

Checklists are just a way to remember tasks. ICU staff have many interventions to perform on a patient in a day. A study found that ICU staff can have up to 178 interactions with a patient in 24 hours, such as giving medication, suctioning, changing sheets, and repositioning. Various experiments conducted by Pollock and Garnerhave shown that the human ability to process information is limited. [20, 21]

44 Intensive Care

Thus, checklists help staff prioritize and avoid missing important tasks. For instance, Pronovost et al conducted a study that reported a significant decrease in the incidence of catheter-related bloodstream infections after introducing a checklist of evidence-based interventions to reduce such infections. The interventions included:

Appropriate hand hygiene, use of chlorhexidine for skin preparation, use of full-barrier precautions during central venous catheter insertion, avoiding femoral site for insertion, and removing unnecessary central venous catheters [22].

A checklist of daily ICU goals during rounds has been shown to improve communication regarding goals of the ICU care among team members [23].

There are four types of checklists described in the literature:

Static parallel checklists are completed by one person and executed as a series of read-and-do tasks. The anesthesia machine checklist is an example.

The static sequential with verification checklist involves a challenge and response. An operator reads a series of items and a second person verifies that each item has been completed or is within parameters. For example, a checklist to ensure the appropriate insertion of a central line.

Static sequential with verification and confirmation checklists are commonly utilized in team-based settings where a group of individuals complete a set of tasks or items. In this format, a designated person reads the items or tasks aloud, and each responsible party confirms the completion of their specific task. This method is frequently used during time-outs and briefings in operating rooms.

The dynamic checklist uses a flowchart to guide complex decision-making. There are multiple options to choose from and the team must decide on the optimal course. An example of a dynamic checklist is the American Society of Anesthesiologists' difficult airway algorithm [24].

However, having too many checklists in the ICU could be counterproductive as staff may find them cumbersome to implement. Therefore, the ICU team leader must identify the processes of care in the units that are prone to human errors or being missed and create a checklist for such activities.

Though evidence-based guidelines are important to provide basic quality of care and reduce variability, one must not forget that medicine is an art. The art component is even more relevant in intensive care where patients suffer from multiple organ dysfunction, have several co-morbidities, and the Intensivist is often faced with complex clinical scenarios.

Outcomes: Measuring the effect of healthcare on the status of the patient is important for quality improvement. The common outcome measures are mortality, length of ICU stay, and quality of life post-ICU stay.

Various quality indicators or key performance indices are used to measure, monitor, and improve the quality of care. The quality indicator used should be relevant to the problem, understandable, measurable (with high dependability and validity), changeable through behavior, achievable, and feasible. For example, to measure the quality of structure, indicators like the nurse-to-patient ratio, doctor-to-patient ratio, nurse attrition rates, and staff burnout are used. To measure the process of care, indicators like ICU infection rates, hand hygiene compliance, medical error rates, use of prophylaxis for prevention of deep vein thrombosis, daily sedation hold, and antibiotic stewardship are used.

Patient and family satisfaction is an important outcome that should be measured. A study was conducted in a Dutch ICU where a tool was created to measure the satisfaction of patients' relatives with the quality of care. The tool consisted of a questionnaire that covered various aspects of the ICU care structure, process, and outcome. The results showed that the most important aspects of care for the family were: no conflicting information, comprehensive information from doctors and nurses, and healthcare professionals taking the patient's relative seriously. The aspects that needed the most urgent improvement were: information about how relatives can contribute to the care of the patient, information about the use of meal facilities in the hospital, and involvement in decision-making on the medical treatment of the patient [25].

The perception of the patient's family may vary from region to region, thus every ICU should attempt to measure family perceptions about the quality of care to make improvements.

Whose responsibility is it to ensure the quality of care?

State, doctors, managers, regulators, accrediting bodies, non-governmental agencies, and patients all have a responsibility to maintain the quality of care. A news article published in 2018 claimed that nearly 5 million deaths are caused by medical errors in India, according to a study conducted by Harvard University. The methodology used to conclude this figure is not known. Nevertheless, it is important to put mechanisms in place to avoid harm due to medical errors.

The state has the responsibility to ensure that all patients receive a basic standard of quality care through various legislations. Regulatory bodies can be appointed by the state to examine the finer details of healthcare provision and scrutinize hospitals against evidence-based standards of quality care.

Doctors and nurses are responsible for the care process in the ICU and should report medical errors and highlight factors that could lead to errors. However, the question is whether they are empowered or protected enough to come forward. Although various medical organizations and literature recommend self-reporting of medical errors as a cornerstone to improving medical care, staff does not report for fear of blame and job loss. Therefore, errors are grossly underreported. Private hospitals do not encourage reporting of medical errors and the factors responsible for them as they may suffer losses. Despite the vast literature on the root cause of medical errors, there is either a lack of understanding or a deliberate attempt to ignore the fact that medical errors are not due to an individual's fault but a failure of the system [26].

For example, an error made by an overworked doctor or nurse is never attributed to the hospital authorities' inability to provide adequate, well-trained staff. It is also not appreciated that the design of the ICU is as crucial as hand hygiene compliance among staff for infection control in the ICU. A system that is vague, disorganized, and unreliable is prone to errors.

In recent years, private hospitals have been hiring hospital managers with a background in business management, giving them the titles of Chief Executive Officer or Chief Operating Officer. These managers are assumed to be responsible for improving the quality of care. However, studies evaluating their impact have produced conflicting results. A systematic review of studies on the role of hospital managers found that senior-level managers spent less than 25% of their time on quality improvement. While some studies reported a positive influence on quality, others reported either no influence or a negative impact on the quality of care [27].

A study was conducted to evaluate the role of managers in non-specialist acute NHS hospitals in England. The study did not find any evidence of an association between quantity of management input and measures of hospital performance like, the proportion of elective patients who are treated within 18 weeks of being referred, the proportion of emergency patients seen within 4 hours, the summary hospital-level mortality indicator and net financial position [28].

Hospital managers employed by the private hospital have the mandate to prioritize profit over quality. Managers who should foster a culture of safety and excellence see healthcare professionals merely as a means to achieve their target of profit. This creates an unhealthy and regressive work environment. Private hospitals in India pay disproportionally higher salaries to certain specialties that bring revenue to the hospitals, which is demoralizing to others and results in poor team effort. Every specialty in the hospital is important to ensure quality care. Such a system of gross pay disparity destroys the holistic concept of healthcare.

There is an interesting study published in The Quarterly Journal of Economics which assessed the moral effects of pay inequality.

48   Intensive Care

The study found that workers reduced output by 52% when their co-workers were paid more than themselves. They were also less likely to come to work, giving up substantial earnings to avoid a workplace where they were paid less than their peers [29].

Privatization of healthcare has altered the concept of quality care. Private hospitals invest in improving aesthetics which instantly pleases patients and their relatives but may not invest in adequate manpower and infrastructure, which is crucial for the safety and quality of patient care. Healthcare services, as a business for profit, may not be good for the health of a society.

Accreditation is a voluntary program sponsored by a non-governmental organization. Trained external peer reviewers evaluate a healthcare organization's compliance and compare it with pre-established performance standards. The American College of Surgeons developed the "Minimum Standard for Hospitals" in 1917. Accreditation began in the United States with the formation of the Joint Commission on Accreditation of Healthcare Organizations (JCAHO) in 1951, and the concept then spread to other parts of the world. Accreditation ensures basic quality standards and professional accountability and encourages healthcare organizations to pursue excellence. There is good evidence that accreditation programs improve the process of care provided by healthcare services, resulting in improved clinical outcomes [30].

But any good idea or intention can be corrupted. What if accrediting bodies indulge in quid pro quo with the hospitals seeking accreditation? Who will monitor the functioning of various accrediting agencies?

Thus, government regulation of hospitals is important if the rights of the patients are to be protected and quality care delivered. For the regulations to be effective, they should be backed by well-informed scientific legislation and, more importantly, have enough resources to implement them. The failure of hospitals to provide quality care is due to a lack of monitoring and the inability of the government to enforce regulations [31].

Finally, patients and the public can provide the strongest stimulus for improved quality of care if they are well-informed and empowered.

This requires disseminating information about diseases, hospital care processes, and hospital performance. For instance, the Leapfrog group is a group of healthcare purchasers in the United States, including 34 members of the Buyers Healthcare Action Group, General Electric, General Motors, GTE, and 45 members of the Pacific Business Group on Health. The Leapfrog group aims to educate and inform consumers about quality healthcare while incentivizing providers by providing them with a business model for quality care.

Patients feel empowered if there is a mechanism for the timely redressal of their complaints.

A systematic review of studies about patient complaints in healthcare found that 33.7% of complaints were quality and safety-related, 35.1% were about management and organization, and 29.1% were patient-staff communication and relationship related [32].

Data from patient complaints can be utilized to enhance the quality and efficiency of healthcare systems. It is recommended that the government make it mandatory for all hospitals to have an online grievance portal for patients and a system to address grievances within a specific timeframe. Since patient complaints offer valuable insights into safety and quality-related concerns, all hospitals should maintain a digital record of complaints that can be easily accessed by regulators to enforce necessary changes for improved quality of care. Numerous studies have shown that patient or family complaints about adverse events in hospitals are reliable [33,34].

A robust patient complaint management system is crucial for transparent and quality healthcare systems.

Sometimes, the quality of care at hospitals can be compromised due to incomplete or patchy services. Critically-ill patients are at risk of developing complications and dysfunction of various organs. If a hospital lacks a particular specialty, the patient may need to be transferred to another hospital, which can be risky and cause delays in receiving definitive treatment. Therefore, it is best for intensive care to be provided at hospitals that have all necessary specialties available.

50   Intensive Care

Quality healthcare requires a concerted effort, and unless all stakeholders exhibit an honest commitment, it may remain elusive.

REFERENCES:

1. Donchin Y, Gopher D, Olin M, et al. A look into the nature and causes of human errors in the intensive care unit. Crit Care Med. 1995; 23(2):294-300.

2. Havens DH, Boroughs L. "To err is human": a report from the Institute of Medicine. Journal of pediatric health care. 2000; 14(2):77-80.

3. Kristensen S, Mainz J, Bartels P. Patient Safety – a Vocabulary for European Application. Aarhus, Denmark: SIMPATIE European Society for Quality in Healthcare – Office for Quality Indicators; 2007.

4. Valentin A, Capuzzo M, Guidet B, et al; Research Group on Quality Improvement of European Society of Intensive Care Medicine; Sentinel Events Evaluation Study Investigators. Patient safety in intensive care: results from the multinational Sentinel Events Evaluation (SEE) study. Intensive Care Med. 2006; 32(10):1591-8.

5. Donchin Y, Gopher D, Olin M, BadihI Y, Biesky MR, Sprung CL, Pizov R, Cotev S. A look into the nature and causes of human errors in the intensive care unit. Critical care medicine. 1995; 23(2):294-300.

6. Bracco D, Favre JB, Bissonnette B, et al. Human errors in a multidisciplinary intensive care unit: a 1-year prospective study. Intensive Care Med. 2001; 27(1):137-45.

7. Donabedian A. The quality of care. How can it be assessed? JAMA. 1988; 260(12):1743-8.

8. Lee HJ, Bae E, Lee HY, Lee SM, Lee J. Association of natural light exposure and delirium according to the presence or absence of windows in the intensive care unit. Acute Crit Care. 2021;36(4):332-341.

9. Smonig R, Magalhaes E, Bouadma L, et al. Impact of natural light exposure on delirium burden in adult patients receiving invasive mechanical ventilation in the ICU: a prospective study. Ann Intensive Care. 2019; 9(1):120.

10. Halaby T, Al NaiemI N, Beishuizen Bet al. Impact of single room design on the spread of multi-drug resistant bacteria in an intensive care unit. Antimicrob Resist Infect Control. 2017; 6:117.

11. Donchin Y, Seagull FJ. The hostile environment of the intensive care unit. CurrOpin Crit Care. 2002; 8(4):316-20.

12. Johnson AL, Brown K, Weaver MT. Sleep deprivation and psychomotor performance among night-shift nurses. AAOHN journal. 2010; 58(4):147-56.

13. Gander P, Purnell H, Garden A, Woodward A. Work patterns and fatigue-related risk among junior doctors. Occup Environ Med. 2007; 64(11):733-8.

14. Smith-Coggins R, Howard SK, Mac DT, et al. Improving alertness and performance in emergency department physicians and nurses: the use of planned naps. Annals of emergency medicine. 2006; 48(5):596-604.

15. Henneman E, Dracup K, Ganz T, et al: Using a collaborative weaning plan to decrease duration of mechanical ventilation and length of stayin the intensive care unit for patients receiving long-term ventilation.Am J Crit Care 2002; 11:132–140.

16. Kollef MH, Shorr A, Tabak YP et al. Epidemiology and outcomes of healthcare associated pneumonia. Chest 2005; 128: 3854–62.

17. Morris AC, Hay AW, SwannDG, et al. Reducing ventilator-associated pneumonia in intensive care: impact of implementing a care bundle. Crit Care Med 2011; 39: 2218–24.

18. Kress JP, Pohlman AS, O'Connor MF, Hall JB: Daily interruption of sedative infusions in critically ill patients undergoing mechanical ventilation. N Engl J Med 2000, 342:1471-1477.

19. Chan PKO, Fischer S, Stewart TE, et al. Practising evidence-based medicine: the design and implementation of a multidisciplinary team-driven extubation protocol. Crit Care. 2001;5:349–354.

20. PollackI. The information of elementary auditory displays. The Journal of the Acoustical Society of America. 1952; 24(6):745-9.

21. Garner WR. An informational analysis of absolute judgments of loudness. Journal of experimental psychology. 1953; 46(5):373.

22. Pronovost P, Needham D, Berenholtz S, et al. An intervention to decrease catheter-related bloodstream infections in the ICU. N Engl J Med. 2006; 355(26):2725-32.

23. Pronovost P, Berenholtz S, Dorman T, Lipsett PA, Simmonds T, Haraden C. Improving communication in the ICU using daily goals. J Crit Care. 2003; 18(2):71-5.

24. Winters BD, Gurses AP, Lehmann H, Sexton JB, Rampersad CJ, Pronovost PJ. Clinical review: checklists - translating evidence into practice. Crit Care. 2009;13(6):210.

25. Rensen A, van Mol MM, Menheere I et al. Quality of care in the intensive care unit from the perspective of patient's relatives: development and psychometric evaluation of the consumer quality index 'R-ICU'. BMC Health Serv Res. 2017; 17(1):77.

26. Bion JF, Heffner JE. Challenges in the care of the acutely ill. Lancet. 2004; 363(9413):970-7.

27. Parand A, Dopson S, Renz A, Vincent C. The role of hospital managers in quality and patient safety: a systematic review. BMJ Open. 2014; 4(9):e005055.

28. Asaria M, McGuire A, Street A. The impact of management on hospital performance. Fiscal Studies. 2022; 43(1):79-95.

29. Breza E, Kaur S, ShamdasanI Y. The morale effects of pay inequality. The Quarterly Journal of Economics. 2018; 133(2):611-63.

30. Alkhenizan A, Shaw C. Impact of accreditation on the quality of healthcare services: a systematic review of the literature. Annals of SaudI medicine. 2011; 31(4):407-16.

31. Muraleedharan VR, Nandraj S. Private health care sector in India: policy challenges and options for partnership. Health Policy Research in South Asia. 2003:229.

32. Reader TW, Gillespie A, Roberts J. Patient complaints in healthcare systems: a systematic review and coding taxonomy. BMJ Qual Saf. 2014; 23(8):678-89.

33. Weingart SN, Pagovich O, Sands DZ, LI JM, Aronson MD, Davis RB, Bates DW, Phillips RS. What can hospitalized patients tell us about adverse events? Learning from patient-reported incidents. J Gen Intern Med. 2005; 20(9):830-6.

34. Agoritsas T, Bovier PA, Perneger TV. Patient reports of undesirable events during hospitalization. J Gen Intern Med. 2005; 20(10):922-8.

CHAPTER 8

RATIONALIZATION OF INTENSIVE CARE

Dr Yogesh Manhas

The cost of intensive care is expensive and it may consume 20% of the total hospital expenditure. The use of new technology in providing life support and the need for highly skilled personnel have raised the cost of ICU care exponentially. Thus, cost effective analysis and rationalizing intensive care is imperative.

Rudolf Virchow, a German pathologist, said, "Politics is medicine on a larger scale," emphasizing the role of social and environmental factors in disease causation and prevention. [1].

The reverse of Rudolf Virchow's statement, "Medicine is politics on a small scale," is partially accurate. Resource allocation is a crucial element of politics, and it is equally important in intensive care medicine. Science and society are interconnected, as science is intended to benefit society. Therefore, ICU leaders must interact with society to understand their expectations of intensive care, educate them about its limitations, and emphasize the dangers of reckless and indiscriminate use of ICU services.

As ICU beds are limited and expensive, intensivists are often faced with the difficult challenge of triaging and prioritizing ICU admissions.

ICU services may be underutilized or misused under different circumstances. Various factors impact the appropriateness of ICU facilities. Let us examine different situations.

A public hospital, funded by taxpayers' money, provides free care to the public. If patients did not have to pay directly out of pocket, there

54 Intensive Care

would be a risk of ICU services being misused given the basis that in many countries there are no clear hospital guidelines and policies legally backed by the state for limiting or withdrawing ICU care when it appears futile.

In the case of private hospitals, patients either pay out of their pocket or have full or limited insurance. Those without insurance may not be able to afford care after a certain time. For instance, a patient with acute respiratory distress syndrome has over a 60% survival chance with quality intensive care, but it may require several weeks of ICU stay with a risk of complications that further increase the cost. Here, the cost becomes a limiting factor, and ICU care may be underutilized. Even those with limited insurance find it challenging to afford costly intensive care at private hospitals. On the other hand, those who can afford it may continue to use ICU services, even when it seems futile regarding the patient's outcome. In countries where healthcare is mainly privatized, there can be significant inequity in intensive care services unless everyone is fully insured.

The aim of rationalizing intensive care is to ensure that any patient who can be saved is given timely intensive care, while patients who are unlikely to benefit from ICU care and have poor outcomes are not admitted.

ICU care is not without complications. The longer the stay in ICU, the greater the risk of complications. Thus, the ICU team needs to set a practical and reasonable goal for ICU care and discuss it with the patient's family. Rationalizing ICU care involves good communication with the patient's family to avoid any unrealistic expectations from family members.

Many intensive care units lack clear admission criteria or policies to limit or withhold ICU care for patients who show no improvement. As a result, ICU beds are occupied by patients on life support with poor long-term prognosis, increasing the cost of care and denying beds to those who could benefit. Continuing life support for patients with poor prognosis can lead to dehumanization and increased suffering, denying patients the dignity to die in peace. Family members suffer from financial burdens, loss of work, lifestyle interference, and loss of quality time with their loved ones.

ICU staff also get frustrated by the continuation of futile ICU care. It reduces morale among them and could lead to burnout.

Patients who are critically ill and on life support have reduced immunity to fight infections, making them highly susceptible to colonization and infection by hospital-acquired organisms. A one-day point prevalence study conducted in European intensive care units revealed that 20.6% of patients had acquired infections while in the ICU [2].

Moreover use of broad spectrum antibiotics in ICU patients increases the development of multidrug-resistant bacteria. These patients then become a reservoir for multidrug-resistant organisms. Continuing life support for patients with a low chance of recovery can contribute to the spread of infections to other patients who have a better chance of being saved.

Trained and experienced intensivists can determine the suitability of intensive care admission. A study was conducted on patients admitted to a tertiary-level ICU in Seoul, where the intensivist's perception was evaluated for beneficial or non-beneficial ICU admission. Patients whose ICU admission was perceived as non-beneficial by intensivists had an 82% in-hospital mortality rate, and none of them survived at the 6-month follow-up [3].

The high cost raises questions about the cost-effectiveness of intensive care. Is it worth the money spent? Does intensive care leave patients dependent with disability? These are important questions for policymakers.

Mortality among patients admitted to the ICU varies widely and depends on several factors, such as the severity of the disease, age, co-morbidities, infrastructure, availability of trained medical staff, nursing care, high or low-intensity staffing patterns in the ICU, hospital-acquired infection rates, etc. The mortality rates in developed

56 Intensive Care

countries range from 9-18%, while mortality is as high as 61% in low-income countries [4].

Several studies have reported on the quality of life in those who survived ICU admission [5-7].

Quality of life in ICU survivors improves over time but remains lower than before their admission to the ICU. A study conducted at the University Hospital in Brussels found that patients who had a prolonged stay in the ICU (>10 days), had a one-year survival rate of 37%. Of the survivors, 27% experienced major functional impairment, while 73% had no or minor physical complaints [8].

Another prospective observational study reported that 38% of the ICU survivors had a worse quality of life than before their ICU admission. 8.3% of the survivors were severely incapacitated [9]. In the same study, 62.2% of patients who worked previously, had returned to work 18 months after ICU discharge.

A cost-effectiveness analysis of ICU care in the NHS UK reported that the incremental cost per quality-adjusted life year gained from treatment in intensive care is £7010, which is well below the threshold incremental cost-effectiveness ratio for NICE approval (i.e. £20,000-£30,000 per quality life adjusted year).

However, the selection of patients for ICU admission is important, and the NHS follows a policy where patients who are too well or too sick to benefit from ICU care are refused admission [10].

The goal of ICU care is not just to prolong life but to add quality to life. It may not be a good outcome if an elderly patient survives but with severe disability and dependence on family members.

"Cost analysis of ICU care can be achieved by a cost block methodology where six cost blocks are identified which are:"

Cost Block 1 includes equipment expenditure.

Cost Block 2 includes maintenance of the ICU structure and utilities.

Cost Block 3 includes Non-Clinical Support Services.

Cost Block 4 includes Clinical Support Services like physiotherapy, radiology, pharmacy, dietetics, and laboratory.

Cost Block 5 includes consumables such as drugs, fluids, nutrition, blood and blood products, and disposables.

Cost Block 6 includes staff salaries of consultants, junior doctors, technicians, and nurses.

Cost analysis conducted using the above method in the UK reported that cost blocks 4 to 6 account for 85% of the ICU cost [11].

Infrastructure, equipment, and staff salaries represent fixed costs, whereas the cost of consumables, pharmacy, laboratory, and radiology is variable. Variable costs depend upon the number of patients admitted, the severity of the disease, length of stay, adherence to evidence-based protocols and policies such as admission and discharge policy, DNR and limitation of care policy, infection control, and antibiotic stewardship.

Several studies suggest that units managed by Intensivists result in better resource utilization with a reduction in variable costs [12-14].

Since staff salaries account for a major portion of ICU cost, it may be tempting to cut costs by reducing the number of staff. However, reducing staff not only compromises the quality of care but may also increase variable costs due to poor ICU resource utilization.

ICU cost reduction can be better achieved by limiting the total number of ICU beds than by reducing staff to manage each ICU bed. Efficiently managed fewer beds fare better than inefficiently managed large number of ICU beds [15].

A systematic review by Pronovost et al demonstrated that high-intensity ICU physician staffing results in reduced ICU and hospital mortality and ICU length of stay [16].

58 Intensive Care

Moreover, a high-intensity staffed intensive care unit is well organized and can handle surges like the recent COVID pandemic much better [17].

Reducing variability in CU care through the use of evidence-based protocols and guidelines can bring down the cost by minimizing unnecessary investigations, procedures, and unproven medical treatment [18].

Infection control and antibiotic stewardship programs reduce costs by decreasing hospital-acquired infections and the associated use of expensive antibiotics to treat infections by multi-drug resistant bacteria.

A clear admission and discharge policy can reduce ICU costs by preventing inappropriate admissions and decreasing delays in ICU discharge [19,20].

However, cost-effective strategies may have different outcomes for different stakeholders and are influenced by a conflict of interest. For example, reducing the length of stay in the ICU is desirable for the patient but may adversely affect private hospital revenue if the ICU beds remains unoccupied.

Similarly, antibiotic stewardship, which is aimed at curtailing the misuse of antibiotics, may bring down pharmacy revenue of a private hospital.

If admissions to the ICU are incentivized by private hospitals, the Intensivist is likely to admit patients who are either too well or too sick to benefit from ICU care. The profit nexus of pharmaceutical companies, private hospitals, and individual doctors can complicate the process of patient care in the ICU. Careful oversight of hospitals by state regulators and insurance companies is required for cost optimization of ICU care. The patients paying out of their pockets are the worst affected by unscrupulous medical practices.

Regionalization of intensive care services can help reduce costs. Regionalization involves the concentration of critical care services at large tertiary referral centers. It is argued that regionalization helps improve outcomes by reducing variability in care as discussed before.

The high volume of patients at referral centers improves the skills and knowledge of care providers, which translates into better outcomes.

Regionalization may minimize the cost of ICU care by reducing the duplication of expensive manpower and infrastructure required for intensive care services at every hospital. Given the scarcity of intensive care-trained manpower across the world, it may not be sustainable to provide a trained 1:1 nurse-patient ratio and intensive care-trained specialists round the clock at every secondary hospital.

However, regionalization has its problems, such as subjecting critically ill patients to the risk of transportation. There may be delays in transferring patients to referral centers. Additionally, since intensive care supports various departments, such as emergency, anesthesia, surgery, etc., the services of these departments may be affected.

Thus, regionalization of intensive care services needs careful planning keeping in mind the geography of the area, robust communication between referring and referral hospitals, well-equipped critical care ambulance and transport staff, and good road infrastructure. The aim is to avoid delays in transportation and ensure continuity of intensive care while transporting the patient to referral centers [21,22].

Regionalization can be combined with telemedicine in intensive care to provide support to secondary hospitals. A systematic review and meta-analysis of eleven observational studies about the effect of telemedicine in intensive care reported reduced ICU mortality and shorter length of stay in ICU when Intensivists were involved through telemedicine in the care of ICU patients. Studies have also reported the cost benefits of telehealth in intensive care [23,24].

Finally, the public can contribute to reducing the cost of ICU by understanding the limitations of intensive care and its futility in terminal illness. Moreover, a significant bulk of ICU admissions are due to the complications of lifestyle diseases like hypertension, diabetes,

60   Intensive Care

obesity, smoking, alcohol/drug abuse, and road traffic accidents which are preventable by awareness and community participation.

REFERENCES:

1. Harden VA. Collected Essays on Public Health and Epidemiology. Resources in the History of Medicine Series No. 1. Cambridge: Science History Publications, 1985:125.

2. Vincent JL, BiharI DJ, Suter PM, et al. The prevalence of nosocomial infection in intensive care units in Europe. Results of the European Prevalence of Infection in Intensive Care (EPIC) Study. EPIC International Advisory Committee. JAMA. 1995; 274(8):639-44.

3. Chang Y, Kim KR, Huh JW, Hong SB, Koh Y, Lim CM. Outcomes of critically ill patients according to the perception of intensivists on the appropriateness of intensive care unit admission. Acute Crit Care. 2021; 36(4):351-360.

4. Abate SM, Assen S, Yinges M, Basu B. Survival and predictors of mortality among patients admitted to the intensive care units in southern Ethiopia: A multi-center cohort study. Ann Med Surg (Lond). 2021; 65:102318.

5. Dowdy DW, Eid MP, Sedrakyan A, Mendez-Tellez PA, Pronovost PJ, Herridge MS, Needham DM. Quality of life in adult survivors of critical illness: a systematic review of the literature. Intensive Care Med. 2005; 31(5):611-20.

6. Hofhuis JGM, Schrijvers AJP, Schermer T, Spronk PE. Health-related quality of life in ICU survivors-10 years later. ScI Rep. 2021; 11(1):15189.

7. Fildissis G, Zidianakis V, Tsigou E, et al. Quality of life outcome of critical care survivors eighteen months after discharge from intensive care. Croat Med J. 2007; 48(6):814-21.

8. RimachI R, Vincent JL, Brimioulle S. Survival and quality of life after prolonged intensive care unit stay. Anaesth Intensive Care. 2007; 35(1):62-7.

9. García Lizana F, Peres Bota D, De Cubber M, Vincent JL. Long-term outcome in ICU patients: what about quality of life?. Intensive care medicine. 2003; 29:1286-93.

10. Ridley S, Morris S. Cost effectiveness of adult intensive care in the UK. Anaesthesia. 2007; 62(6):547-54.

11. Edbrooke D, Hibbert C, Ridley S, Long T, Dickie H. The development of a method for comparative costing of individual intensive care units. Anaesthesia 1999; 54: 110–20.

12. Multz AS, Chalfin DB, Samson IM, Dantzker DR, Fein AM, Steinberg HN, Niederman MS, Scharf SM. A "closed" medical intensive care unit (MICU) improves resource utilization when compared with an "open" MICU. Am J Respir Crit Care Med. 1998 May;157(5 Pt 1):1468-73.

13. Pronovost P, Angus DC. Economics of managing death in the ICU. In: Curtis JR, Rubenfeld GD, editors. Managing death in the ICU: the transition from cure to comfort. New York: Oxford University Press; 2001. p. 245–255.

14. Kollef MH, Ward S. The influence of access to a private attending physician on the withdrawal of life-sustaining therapies in the intensive care unit. Crit Care Med 1999;27:2125–2132.

15. Valley TS, NoritomI DT. ICU beds: less is more? Yes. Intensive Care Med. 2020; 46(8):1594-1596.

16. Pronovost PJ, Angus DC, Dorman T, Robinson KA, Dremsizov TT, Young TL. Physician staffing patterns and clinical outcomes in critically ill patients: a systematic review. JAMA. 2002; 288(17):2151-62.

17. ArabI YM, Azoulay E, Al-DorzI HM, et al. How the COVID-19 pandemic will change the future of critical care. Intensive Care Med. 2021; 47(3):282-291.

18. Kahn JM, Angus DC. Reducing the cost of critical care: new challenges, new solutions. Am J Respir Crit Care Med. 2006; 174(11):1167-8.

19. Masoompour SM, Askarian M, NajibI M, Hatam N. The financial burden of inappropriate admissions to intensive care units of Shahid FaghihI and Nemazee Hospitals of Shiraz, Iran, 2014. Shiraz E-Medical Journal. 2016; 17(11).

20. Bagshaw SM, Tran DT, Opgenorth D, Wang X, Zuege DJ, Ingolfsson A, Stelfox HT, Thanh NX. Assessment of Costs of Avoidable Delays in Intensive Care Unit Discharge. JAMA Netw Open. 2020 ;3(8):e2013913.

21. Singh JM, MacDonald RD. Pro/con debate: do the benefits of regionalized critical care delivery outweigh the risks of interfacility patient transport? Crit Care. 2009;13(4):219.

22. Suntharalingam G, Handy J, Walsh A. Regionalisation of critical care: can we sustain an intensive care unit in every hospital? Anaesthesia. 2014 Oct;69(10):1069-73.

23. Wilcox ME, AdhikarI NK. The effect of telemedicine in critically ill patients: systematic review and meta-analysis. Crit Care. 2012; 16(4):R127.

24. Cole S, Robie M, Abodunde B, Coustasse A. Telehealth in Critical Care: Quality and Cost Outcomes. Proceedings of the Northeast Business & Economics Association 2019 Conference (pp. 245-252).

CHAPTER 9

DO NOT RESUSCITATE (DNR), WITHHOLDING AND WITHDRAWAL OF CARE

(END OF LIFE DECISIONS)

Dr Abhijit Nair/ Dr Yogesh Manhas

Intensive care provides support to the organs affected by illnesses until the severity of the illness becomes less or is cured by definitive treatment. However, intensive care may not be able to achieve the desired outcome in terminal organ failure.

The question to be asked is whether a terminally ill patient would like to die peacefully in the comfort of their home in the presence of family members or in the ICU surrounded by unfamiliar faces of doctors and nurses who, out of professional obligation, frantically push on the chest trying to get a few days, hours, or just minutes of life back in the event of cardiac arrest.

A public opinion poll conducted by Gallup in the USA reported that 9 out of 10 people would prefer to be cared for at home if they were terminally ill with six months or less to live [1]. However, there is a consistent rise in the number of patients who end up in intensive care units in the last few days of their lives. An analysis of all deaths from six large states in the USA found that one in five people died in intensive care units [2].

Advanced cardiovascular life support (ACLS) protocols are useful in saving lives, but their usefulness in terminally ill patients and those on life support with little chance of recovery is questionable. To avoid futile efforts of cardiopulmonary resuscitation and prolonging the suffering of a dying patient, do-not-resuscitate (DNR) orders are activated. DNR means not attempting resuscitation in the event of cardiopulmonary arrest. DNR does not mean that the patient will not receive treatment, nor does it mean that the patient will be abandoned and not cared for.

However, DNR may not serve its purpose when the patient is already on life support measures, in which case withholding and/or withdrawal of care need to be considered. Withholding means not escalating treatment, while withdrawal involves the removal of therapy meant to sustain life. Decisions for DNR, withholding, or withdrawal of therapy should follow four basic principles of ethics:

Autonomy: The patient's wishes to accept or refuse treatment must be respected.

Beneficence: Provide benefits in the best interest of the individual patient, balancing benefits and risks.

Non-maleficence: No therapy should prolong suffering. Do no harm.

Justice: In this context, it's about the rationing of ICU beds. Blocking an ICU bed by continuing futile therapy may keep a salvageable patient bereft of ICU care.

A futile therapy or intervention is one that is unlikely to restore, maintain, or enhance a life that the patient can be aware of [3]. However, there are controversies concerning the definition of medical futility [4]. Schneiderman and colleagues define futility as the desired outcome, although possible, being overwhelmingly improbable [5].

DNR, withholding, and withdrawal of care are end-of-life decisions that should be made with great sensitivity and close communication with family members. These decisions are influenced by the cultural and religious practices of both the caregiver and the patient and their family members [6]. Being aware of the patient's cultural and religious sentiments helps to create trust between the caregiver and the patient's family.

DNR orders are activated in a critically ill patient by the primary physician or intensivist involved in the patient's care after a discussion with the patient or their surrogate decision-maker. These decisions are tough, and the conversation between the two parties involved could vary depending on the circumstances and the patient's condition [7]. Critically ill patients may be unconscious, under the influence of ongoing sedation, or unable to make decisions due to advanced age or underlying medical conditions such as electrolyte imbalances or other metabolic derangements.

The acceptance of DNR by the patient and/or family member is influenced by various factors, such as their understanding of the underlying disease, educational status, previous experiences with family or friends, and inability to make such a significant decision alone. Some family members believe that DNR is the same as passive euthanasia, so they either do not agree or postpone the decision due to indecisiveness [8]. Chu and Hynes-Gay's review article concluded that there is no proof that patients whose DNR status is activated are abandoned in any way [9].

Therefore, DNR orders should not be imposed on patients. The decision maker should be allowed sufficient time to contemplate and make a decision. Some family members view DNR as a termination of treatment, resulting in the patient receiving inadequate or no care at all. However, they must be assured that supportive care, such as feeding, ongoing pain relief medication, bowel care, and chest and limb physiotherapy, will persist despite DNR orders.

FACTORS INFLUENCING DNR ACTIVATION:

The factors that may affect DNR activation can be attributed to either the physician or the patient/family member. Physician-related factors include medico-legal concerns, insufficient understanding of palliative care principles, or a desire to pursue aggressive treatment regardless of the patient's condition. Additionally, a busy schedule for the treating team has been identified as a potential cause for hesitation in discussing DNR options for patients [10,11].

The patient/family factors responsible are fear, lack of knowledge and understanding, and religious and cultural issues which prohibit them from consenting to DNR. The discussion on DNR should not be abandoned if the family members do not agree in the first meeting with the treating team. Whenever updates are provided to them about the patient's condition, the discussion can be reinitiated again. Sometimes a change in the person initiating the discussion is advisable.

TIMING OF DNR ORDERS:

There is no specific timing for DNR orders. Once the critical care team becomes involved and determines that aggressive treatment is not justified due to the advanced nature of the disease, DNR orders can be put into effect. Shiu et al conducted a retrospective study of 386 patients and stressed the importance of documenting and activating DNR status early to prevent chest compression, DC shock administration, and the use of cardiotonic drugs in terminally ill patients [12].

In another study by Ouyang et al, the authors enrolled 200 patients and 83 nurses taking care of critically ill patients admitted to a medical ICU and cardiac ICU and interviewed their perceptions on the patient's quality of death [13]. On analysis, they concluded that activating DNR orders within the first 48 hours of ICU admission was associated with fewer non-beneficial procedures, less suffering, lesser loss of dignity, and lower odds of being not at peace and of having the worst possible death.

On many occasions, patients arrive at the emergency room in a sick state that requires endotracheal intubation and mechanical ventilation. Some clinicians believe that a DNR order would have been appropriate in this situation and that the intubation was unnecessary. However, DNR orders can still be placed while mechanical ventilation is ongoing. The plan should be to keep the patient comfortable and avoid invasive procedures and unnecessary investigations, including imaging [14].

The overall workload of the critical unit has been identified as a factor responsible for hindering the activation of DNR. In a retrospective, observational study by Lin et al, the authors concluded that physicians with heavier workloads, indicated by caring for more

66   Intensive Care

patients per day, were less likely to write a DNR order. This could be due to time-consuming counseling sessions, documentation, and legal hassles that could affect the decision-making process [15].

Such situations can be addressed by emphasizing the importance and concept of DNR to hospital management. Once in the loop, hospital management can appoint dedicated personnel such as the nursing in charge, the public relation officer, or someone else who could be the focal point in such situations.

ARE SURGERIES/INTERVENTIONS ALLOWED IN DNR STATUS?

Patients admitted to the hospital with DNR status pose unique situations that raise difficult queries. Imagine a DNR patient with terminal malignancy who presents with an acute intestinal obstruction or perforation unrelated to the disease that led to DNR orders and now requires surgical intervention. Other examples include the need for a tracheostomy, debridement for bed sores, percutaneous gastrostomy tube (PEG) placement, invasive vascular access, and more. The ethical question arising here is whether these interventions can be performed with the DNR orders active or whether the DNR order needs to be made inactive and reactivated once the procedure is over [16].

Just like cardiopulmonary resuscitation, any surgery proposed in a DNR patient is an intervention. In a perioperative setting, there is not enough clarity on whether such patients should be accepted for surgery or not. Surgeries in terminally ill DNR patients are usually palliative or proposed to make the situation comfortable. For example, a tracheostomy will facilitate weaning from a mechanical ventilator, a PEG tube placement will facilitate feeding, a chest tube could relieve respiratory embarrassment, and an invasive line could be used to provide adequate comfort in the form of opioids and sedation. Many hospitals temporarily suspend the DNR orders until the intervention is performed and then reactivate it. This clause is controversial as many feel that deactivating DNR, although temporary, is a violation of the patient's autonomy, who has already accepted and desired DNR status. Hospitals need to have unique policies for such unusual situations. The pros and cons of the intervention need to be discussed with the patient and/or family members, and the procedure involved (deactivation and reactivation of DNR) needs to be informed to them [17].

DNR PATIENT IN THE ICU:

Though a patient with a DNR order can technically still receive ICU care, they are often deemed unsuitable for admission. Therefore, it is crucial to discuss limiting or withholding certain medical care, including ICU admission, when discussing the DNR issue with the patient's family. Admitting a critically ill patient with DNR orders to the ICU presents numerous challenges, including high costs for the hospital and patient, taking up a bed that could be used for a salvageable patient, and requiring significant time and effort from medical staff.

Formal training and knowledge of palliative care practices are essential in determining the timing of DNR by the intensivist. The decision-making process can be difficult for the patient care team due to ethical considerations and multiple clinical dilemmas, which can result in delays in activating DNR [18,19].

Across the world, there is wide variability in the application of End of Life decisions. There is no universal consensus on how these decisions are to be made and implemented [20].

A systematic review on end-of-life decisions found that the prevalence of treatment withdrawal ranged from 0 to 84% in different studies, while treatment withholding varied from 5.3% to 67.3%. This variability was observed not only between countries but also within a country and among different intensive care units. While withholding and withdrawal of treatment are considered ethically equivalent in the West, this is not the case in Asia and the Middle East [21]. A study examining end-of-life decision-making practices in Asian intensive care units revealed that nearly 70% of respondents reported withholding treatment, while only 20% reported withdrawing treatment [22].

68   Intensive Care

Jean-Louis Vincent, Professor of Intensive Care Medicine at the University of Brussels, has convincingly argued why life support measures should be withdrawn when they no longer benefit the patient [23]. He believes that not withdrawing therapy would go against the four basic principles of ethics: it would strip the patient of their autonomy, provide no benefit to the patient, prolong suffering, and prevent a salvageable patient from receiving the benefits of ICU care. Additionally, he argues that allowing withdrawal makes physicians more willing to give a trial of ICU care when there is uncertainty about the benefits of ICU care and the patient's prognosis. Knowing that life support can be withdrawn if the trial of ICU fails prevents delays and indecisiveness in instituting intensive care.

Much of the variability in end-of-life decisions is due to cultural, religious, geographical, and historical factors. Moreover, the lack of adequate legislation is a big hindrance not only in providing end-of-life care but also in the efficient utilization of scarce ICU resources.

To conclude, activating DNR status is an important aspect of patient care. The comfort care offered to these patients reduces futile interventions, saves time, keeps the patient pain-free, and creates a bed for a salvageable patient. The patient and family members need to be explained in detail about the plan of care, and proper documentation needs to be done once agreed upon.

REFERENCES:

1. Fields MJ, Cassel CK: Approaching Death, Improving Care at the End of Life. Washington DC, National Academy Press, 1997.

2. Angus DC, Barnato AE, Linde-Zwirble WT, et al; Robert Wood Johnson Foundation ICU End-Of-Life Peer Group. Use of intensive care at the end of life in the United States: an epidemiologic study. Crit Care Med. 2004; 32(3):638-43.

3. Ravitsky V, Fiester A, Caplan AL, editors. The Penn Center guide to bioethics. Springer Publishing Company; 2009 Apr 16.

4. Bernat JL. Medical futility: definition, determination, and disputes in critical care. Neurocrit Care. 2005;2(2):198-205.

5. Schneiderman LJ, Jecker NS, Jonsen AR. Medical futility: itsmeaning and ethical implications. Ann Intern Med 1990;112:949–954.

6. Manalo MF. End-of-Life Decisions about Withholding or Withdrawing Therapy: Medical, Ethical, and Religio-Cultural Considerations. Palliat Care. 2013; 7:1-5.

7. Downar J, Luk T, Sibbald RW, SantinI T, Mikhael J, Berman H, Hawryluck L. Why do patients agree to a "Do not resuscitate" or "Full code" order? Perspectives of medical inpatients. J Gen Intern Med. 2011; 26(6):582-7.

8. AnnaduraI K, Danasekaran R, ManI G. 'Euthanasia: right to die with dignity'. J Family Med Prim Care. 2014; 3(4):477-8.

9. Chu W, Hynes-Gay P. The influence of DNR orders on patient care in adult ICUs: a review of the evidence. Dynamics. 2002 Winter;13(4):14-21.

10. (Tanuseputro P, Hsu A, Chalifoux M, et al. Do-Not-Resuscitate and Do-Not-Hospitalize Orders in Nursing Homes: Who Gets Them and Do They Make a Difference? J Am Med Dir Assoc. 2019 Sep;20(9):1169-1174.)

11. Lin KH, Huang SC, Wang CH, Chau-Chung, Chu TS, Chen YY. Physician workload associated with do-not-resuscitate decision-making in intensive care units: an observational study using Cox proportional hazards analysis. BMC Med Ethics. 2019; 20(1):15.

12. Shiu SS, Lee TT, Yeh MC, Chen YC, Huang SH. The Impact of Signing Do-Not-Resuscitate Orders on the Use of Non-Beneficial Life-Sustaining Treatments for Intensive Care Unit Patients: A Retrospective Study. Int J Environ Res Public Health. 2022; 19(15):9521.

13. Ouyang DJ, Lief L, Russell D, et al. Timing is everything: Early do-not-resuscitate orders in the intensive care unit and patient outcomes. PLoS One. 2020; 15(2):e0227971.

14. Chang Y, Huang CF, Lin CC. Do-not-resuscitate orders for critically ill patients in intensive care. Nurs Ethics. 2010; 17(4):445-55.

15. Lin KH, Huang SC, Wang CH, Chau-Chung, Chu TS, Chen YY. Physician workload associated with do-not-resuscitate decision-making in intensive care units: an observational study using Cox proportional hazards analysis. BMC Med Ethics. 2019;20(1):15.

16. Hiestand D, Beaman M. Perioperative Do-Not-Resuscitate Suspension: The Patient's Perspective. AORN J. 2019;109(3):326-334.

17. Kushelev M, Meyers LD, Palettas M, et al. Perioperative do-not-resuscitate orders: Trainee experiential learning in preserving patient autonomy and knowledge of professional guidelines. Medicine (Baltimore). 2021;100(11):e24836.

18. Sulmasy DP, He MK, McAuley R, Ury WA. Beliefs and attitudes of nurses and physicians about do not resuscitate orders and who should speak to patients and families about them. Crit Care Med. 2008; 36(6):1817-22.

19. Connolly C, MiskolcI O, Phelan D, Buggy DJ. End-of-life in the ICU: moving from 'withdrawal of care' to palliative care, patient-centered approach. Br J Anaesth. 2016; 117(2):143-5.

20. Santonocito C, Ristagno G, Gullo A, Weil MH. Do-not-resuscitate order: a view throughout the world. J Crit Care. 2013 Feb;28(1):14-21.

21. Mark NM, Rayner SG, Lee NJ, Curtis JR. Global variability in withholding and withdrawal of life-sustaining treatment in the intensive care unit: a systematic review. Intensive Care Med. 2015; 41(9):1572-85.

22. Phua J, Joynt GM, Nishimura M, et al; ACME Study Investigators and the Asian Critical Care Clinical Trials Group. Withholding and withdrawal of life-sustaining treatments in intensive care units in Asia. JAMA Intern Med. 2015; 175(3):363-71.

23. Vincent JL. Withdrawing may be preferable to withholding. Crit Care. 2005; 9(3):226-9.

CHAPTER 10

PEACEFUL TRANSITION FROM LIFE TO DEATH

Dr Yogesh Manhas

With the availability of intensive care services, many patients breathe their last in intensive care units. In America, 20% of deaths occur in intensive care units (ICU). In India, approximately 10–36% of patients admitted to the ICU die. A study conducted in a German tertiary hospital over two years reported 37% of deaths in ICUs [1-3].

Thus, it is incumbent upon the intensivist to use all possible means available to ensure that the patient does not die in distress and discomfort. Death can be a good outcome when medical therapies become futile and no meaningful outcome can be achieved. Life support therapies are not meant to prolong suffering. Once end of life decisions are made, it is the responsibility of the ICU team to ensure that the patient dies peacefully without experiencing any pain. Equally important is that family understand and accept the decision without any apprehensions or guilt. Therefore, maintaining close communication with family members is important in such situations.

The Institute of Medicine defines the quality of death as "a death that is free from avoidable distress and suffering for patients, families, and their caregivers; in general accord with the patient's and families wishes; and reasonably consistent with clinical, cultural, and ethical standards [4]."

However, the quality of death is difficult to attain. The SUPPORT study revealed deficiencies in end-of-life care for critically ill patients. Only 47% of doctors were aware of the patient's wish to avoid CPR.

72   Intensive Care

Nearly 50% of patients who expressed a desire to withhold CPR did not have a DNR order documented during their hospital stay. According to interviews with families, 50% of conscious patients who passed away experienced moderate to severe pain for at least half the time of their last three days of life [5].

Donald L Patrick et al. proposed a model for evaluating the quality of death. They generated six conceptual domains consisting of 31 aspects that patients can rate according to their importance before death. Later, families and clinicians can assess these aspects after death to evaluate the quality of the dying experience. The authors relied on prior literature on the dying experience and conducted qualitative interviews with people with and without terminal illnesses to develop this model [6].

The six domains and their aspects are as follows:

Symptoms and personal care:

1. Having pain under control
2. Having control over what is going on around you
3. Being able to feed oneself
4. Having control of the urinary bladder, bowels
5. Being able to breathe comfortably
6. Having the energy to do things one wants to do

Preparation for Death

1. Feeling at peace with dying
2. Feeling unafraid of dying
3. Avoiding strain on loved ones.
4. Having healthcare costs covered.
5. Having visits from a religious leader
6. Having a spiritual service or ceremony before death.
7. Having funeral arrangements in order.
8. Saying goodbye to loved ones.
9. Attending important events.
10. Clearing up bad feelings

Moment of Death

1. Dying in the place of one's choice
2. Dying in the state of one's choice (i.e., asleep, awake, or unconscious).
3. Having desired people present at the time of one's death

Family

1. Spending time with spouse/partner.
2. Spending time with children.
3. Spending time with family, friends
4. Spending time alone.
5. Spending time with pets.

Treatment Preferences

1. Have discussed end-of-life wishes with your doctor
2. Avoid using a ventilator or dialysis
3. Have the means to end life if desired

Whole Person Concerns

1. Being able to laugh and smile
2. Being touched and hugged.
3. Finding meaning and purpose
4. Keeping one's dignity and self-respect.

The difficulty is that it is not always possible to identify dying patients in advance given the prognostic uncertainty. Moreover, at the time or a few days before death, the patient may be incompetent to inform about their preferences. In certain situations, it may not be possible to consider a particular preference due to constraints beyond control in the ICU setting. However, whenever patients can make their preferences known and if feasible, they should be respected.

An advance directive is a living will that states a person's preferences for medical treatment should they become incapacitated and unable to make decisions during their illness. Advance directives aid in advance care planning. A multidisciplinary DelphI panel describes advance care planning as a process that ensures people receive medical care that is consistent with their values, goals, and preferences during serious and chronic illness [7].

A systematic review of studies identified six goals of advanced care planning [8]:

Respecting individual patient autonomy.

Improving the quality of care.

Strengthening relationships.

Preparing for end-of-life.

Reducing overtreatment.

Though advance directives and advance care planning intend to improve end-of-life care, there are several studies indicating that advance directives are not implemented in practice [9-11].

The problem with advance directives is that very few patients have them when they become critically ill, as many end up in the ICU without warning. With the exception of those with malignancies, most people do not want to consider their own death and are not familiar with various ICU care processes. Many patients rely on their families to make decisions for them during severe illness. Additionally, a person's level of education and religious beliefs can influence whether they have an advance directive or not. Physicians may sometimes not respect advance directives due to a lack of clarity about treatment options in the document. Advance directives may not cover all possible scenarios that may arise during illness, and physicians may be concerned about potential litigation from the family.

Whether there is an advance directive or not, once ICU treatment seems futile with no meaningful outcome for the patient, intensivists should hold a family counseling session. This session should not only inform them about the poor prognosis but also explore their expectations from ICU care and the patient's values and beliefs. When it comes to decision-making, a shared approach may be better than a paternalistic one. A shared approach provides information to the families about the patient, respects their opinion, makes recommendations, and helps them reach a decision. Decision-making on behalf of a dying patient is a huge burden and can lead to conflict among family members. It is a good exercise to ask yourself, "How would I be feeling in this particular situation?" to understand the ordeal of the families.[12].

A study was conducted in 22 French intensive care units where end-of-life counseling with the family was based on five objectives summarized by the mnemonic VALUE: Value and appreciate what the family members said, Acknowledge the family members' emotions, Listen, Ask questions that would allow the caregiver to understand who the patient was as a person, and Elicit questions from the family members. The study reported that using the VALUE communication format resulted in decreased post-traumatic stress disorder, anxiety, and depression among families after the death of their loved one in the ICU [13].

The behavior of the Intensivist should always enhance patient dignity. During family counseling, they should demonstrate how patients and their families are important to them. Not rushing, listening patiently, and making eye contact when talking instill reassurance among family members that their patients shall be taken care of well [14]. Harvey Chochinov describes ABCD of dignity-conserving care referring to the importance of **Attitude, Behavior, Compassion,** and **Dialogue** while caring for a dying patient.

Death and spirituality are closely linked, and it is during the dying moment when one seeks spirituality the most. Thus, being aware of the local culture and spiritual beliefs of the patient and their family helps to provide better end-of-life care.

Once a shared decision with the family is made to forego life support therapies, the goal of ICU care changes from cure to comfort care.

76 Intensive Care

Every member of the ICU team, as well as the primary physician/ surgeon, is made aware of the plan. Family members should be explained about various therapies that shall be withheld or withdrawn and the resulting consequences. They should also be informed that the use of some medications for comfort care may hasten the process of dying. Unnecessary devices, equipment, and medications should be removed. Only those medications that are necessary to ensure the comfort of the patient (analgesics, sedatives, laxatives) are continued.

In no case should the family ever feel that the patient is being abandoned. Let family members stay with the patient and provide them with comfortable chairs at the bedside. Allow them to carry out any rituals that are feasible in the ICU setting.

The Consensus for Worldwide End-of-Life Practice for Patients in Intensive Care Units (WELPICUS) is a study that sought responses about end-of-life practices from critical care societies in 32 countries. Based on the consensus, it published definitions and statements regarding end-of-life practices in intensive care [15].

End-of-life care is a quality improvement index in many intensive care units, requiring compassion, patience, and sensitivity from the ICU team. The comfort and dignity of the dying patient, as well as the satisfaction of their family, is a fine art of intensive care medicine.

REFERENCES:

1. Angus DC, Barnato AE, Linde-Zwirble WT, et al; Robert Wood Johnson Foundation ICU End-Of-Life Peer Group. Use of intensive care at the end of life in the United States: an epidemiologic study. Crit Care Med. 2004;32(3):638-43.

2. Parikh CR, Karnad DR. Quality, cost and outcome of intensive care in a public hospital in Bombay. Crit Care Med 1999;27:1754-9.

3. Ay E, Weigand MA, Röhrig R, Gruss M. Dying in the Intensive Care Unit (ICU): A Retrospective Descriptive Analysis of Deaths in the ICU in a Communal Tertiary Hospital in Germany. Anesthesiol Res Pract. 2020;2020:2356019.

4. Field MJ, Cassell CK, eds. Approaching death: improving care at the end of life. Washington, DC: National Academy Press, 1997.

5. A controlled trial to improve care for seriously ill hospitalized patients. The study to understand prognoses and preferences for outcomes and risks of treatments (SUPPORT). The SUPPORT Principal Investigators. JAMA. 1995;274(20):1591-8. Erratum in: JAMA 1996;275(16):1232.

6. Patrick DL, Engelberg RA, Curtis JR. Evaluating the quality of dying and death. J Pain Symptom Manage. 2001;22(3):717-26.

7. Sudore RL, Lum HD, You JJ, et al. Defining Advance Care Planning for Adults: A Consensus Definition From a Multidisciplinary DelphI Panel. J Pain Symptom Manage. 2017; 53:821–32.e1.

8. Fleuren N, Depla MFIA, Janssen DJA, Huisman M, Hertogh CMPM. Underlying goals of advance care planning (ACP): a qualitative analysis of the literature. BMC Palliat Care. 2020;19(1):27.

9. Halpern NA, Pastores SM, Chou JF, Chawla S, Thaler HT. Advance directives in an oncologic intensive care unit: a contemporary analysis of their frequency, type, and impact. J Palliat Med. 2011;14(4):483-9.

10. Westphal DM, McKee SA. End-of-life decision making in the intensive care unit: physician and nurse perspectives. Am J Med Qual. 2009; 24:222-228.

11. Danis M, Southerland LI, Garrett JM, et al. A prospective study of advance directives for life-sustaining care. N Engl J Med. 1991;324(13):882 8.

12. Azoulay E, Pochard F, Kentish-BarnesN, et al. Risk of post-traumatic stress symptoms in family members of intensive care unit patients. Am J Respir Crit Care Med 2005; 171:987-94.

13. Lautrette A, Darmon M, Megarbane B, et al. A communication strategy and brochure for relatives of patients dying in the ICU. N Engl J Med. 2007;356(5):469-78.

14. Chochinov HM. Dignity and the essence of medicine: the A, B, C, and D of dignity conserving care. BMJ. 2007;335(7612):184-7.

15. Sprung CL, Truog RD, Curtis JR, et al. Seeking worldwide professional consensus on the principles of end-of-life care for the critically ill. The Consensus for Worldwide End-of-Life Practice for Patients in Intensive Care Units (WELPICUS) study. Am J Respir Crit Care Med. 2014;190(8):855-66.

CHAPTER 11

POST-INTENSIVE CARE REHABILITATION

Dr. Yogesh Manhas

Survivors of critical illness suffer from a variety of problems post-discharge from the intensive care unit. Critical illness and prolonged immobility have profound changes in patients' organs that affect their daily activities. There is deconditioning of the respiratory, cardiovascular, and neuromuscular systems. Muscles get atrophied and weak, and there are adverse changes in the cardiovascular and respiratory system that blunt the normal reflex and compensatory mechanisms. During ICU stay, patients may develop critical illness myopathy, neuropathy, and muscle deconditioning, collectively called Intensive care unit-acquired weakness. The more severe the illness, the greater the chances of developing critical myopathy/neuropathy. Patients may also suffer from sleeplessness, nightmares, loss of appetite, anxiety, depression, cognitive impairment, sexual dysfunction, visual impairment, muscle weakness, chronic fatigue syndrome, etc. These post-ICU problems are grouped as Post intensive care syndrome (PICS) [1].

Several risk factors for ICU-acquired weakness are sepsis, female sex, multiorgan failure, prolonged mechanical ventilation, high blood sugar, use of steroids, and paralyzing agents.

In a study involving survivors of acute respiratory distress syndrome (ARDS), physical limitations persisted up to 5 years post-ICU discharge [2].

Cognitive impairment is common in ICU survivors. Studies have reported an incidence of 30-80% [3].

Cognitive impairment is not only disabling for patients but also causes stress for their families. Patients with cognitive impairment may experience memory loss, difficulty understanding, concentrating, and completing tasks. They may also have mood changes and be unaware of their surroundings at times. ICU delirium is one of the most significant risk factors associated with cognitive impairment [4]. The longer the duration of ICU delirium, the higher the risk of cognitive impairment.

Delirium can be hypoactive, where patients are calm but do not think clearly and are inattentive. Others are agitated and combative, called hyperactive delirium. Some patients fluctuate between these two types. Hypoactive delirium is easily missed. However, it is more common than hyperactive, especially in older patients. What causes delirium is not clear, but there is a strong association with the use of long-acting benzodiazepines used as sedatives in the ICU [5].

Other factors associated with cognitive impairment are wide fluctuations in blood sugar, hypoxemia, hypotension, and the use of sedatives.

Psychological disturbances include symptoms of anxiety, depression, and sleep disturbances. According to research, 30% of ICU survivors experience symptoms of depression, while up to 50% develop anxiety [6].

A meta-analysis reported symptoms of post-traumatic stress disorder in one-fifth of ICU survivors at one-year follow-up [7].

PICS affects not only patients who have survived intensive care, but also their families, known as PICS-F. Studies have shown that anxiety affects up to 10-75% of patients' families. Approximately 33% of family members of the patient experience post-traumatic stress disorder, and this number is even higher if the patient is a child or did not survive [8-10].

PICS cause a significant financial burden on the family as 50% of the patients do not return to work one year post-discharge and 30% never return to work. 20% of family members may have to leave their employment to care for the ICU survivors [11].

80   Intensive Care

Though PICS is mentioned in the literature, unfortunately it is not given the attention it deserves in clinical practice. The ICU team's efforts to save critically ill patients are overshadowed by the serious impairment of lives post-discharge due to physical and mental disabilities. PICS is not routinely discussed or considered during daily rounds of ICU patients, nor is it a common topic of discussion at intensive care conferences. The point is that PICS requires as much attention as the acute illness for which the patient was admitted to the ICU.

A solution to any problem starts with its acknowledgment. Every ICU team member, as well as other specialties, needs to be sensitized to PICS, a problem that requires a multidisciplinary approach. Patients and family members should be counseled regarding PICS while the patient is recovering in ICU. It may be a good idea to get the patient evaluated by a physiotherapist, respiratory therapist, occupational therapist, speech therapist, and psychologist/psychiatrist to assess patient needs and advise follow-up before they are discharged from ICU. This would provide an estimate of problems that need to be addressed and help prepare patients, family members, and concerned specialties for future courses of action.

The Society of Critical Care Medicine took action to raise awareness about PICS by organizing a stakeholder conference in both 2010 and 2012. The stakeholders in attendance were representatives from national noncritical care organizations, including the Joint Commission, National Institutes of Health, primary care, rehabilitation, physical therapy, occupational therapy, speech-language-hearing, long-term care, palliative care, case workers, patients, families, and patient advocacy groups [12,13].

The Society of Critical Care Medicine awards grants of up to $50,000 to members who conduct research aimed at improving patient and family support and recovery after critical illness through an initiative called "Thrive" [14].

Critical care societies in various countries across the world need to take initiatives to spread awareness and conduct research to improve the quality of life in ICU survivors.

What has been done so far and what are the strategies to reduce PICS in ICU survivors?

EARLY MOBILIZATION AND PHYSICAL REHABILITATION:

Early mobilization of ICU patients improves muscle strength and decreases ICU and hospital length of stay. It also improves the mobility and functional status of the patient [15].

Studies have shown that early physical rehabilitation decreases the chances of ICU-acquired weakness [16].

Physical rehabilitation for mobility involves activities such as sitting at the edge of the bed, standing, ambulation, and passive exercises including range-of-motion exercises. It can be initiated as soon as the patient is stable enough. These activities can be performed safely while the patient is connected to mechanical ventilators and monitors. The presence of catheters and lines does not preclude early physical rehabilitation [17].

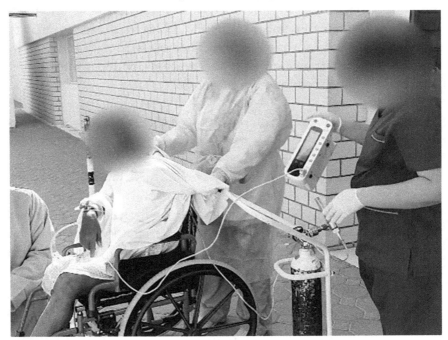

Mobilizing ICU patient in a wheelchair.

82 Intensive Care

ABCDEFGH Bundle: The bundle is designed to remind healthcare providers of interventions that can reduce risk factors for PICS while caring for patients in the ICU.

A- Assess, prevent, and manage pain.
B- Breathing trials, daily interruption of sedation followed by a spontaneous breathing trial.
C- Choice of analgesia and sedation, coordination of care, and communication.
D- Delirium assessment, prevention, and management.
E- Early mobility.
F- Family involvement, follow-up referrals, and functional reconciliation.
G- Good handoff communication among nurses between shifts..
H- Handout materials on PICS and PICS-F.

Functional reconciliation is a concept that involves comparing a patient's current functional status with their status before hospitalization. When a patient arrives at the hospital, an initial assessment of their functional status should be conducted, similar to the assessment done for medications. This assessment should then be reconciled at each transition within institutions, between institutions, and with outpatient/community resources.

Functional reconciliation requires close collaboration between nurses and therapists.

Intensive care unit diaries are kept by families and staff to describe the patient's experience and record the patient's status while in the ICU. Diaries are written by a caring nurse or a family member. Sometimes pictures are included in the diaries. Doctors, respiratory therapists, and physiotherapists can also add to the diaries. Diaries are useful for the patient when discharged to fill memory gaps, understand what happened to them, and remove false memories. They can prevent PICS by decreasing anxiety, depression, and post-traumatic stress disorder [18].

Diaries have also been shown to decrease symptoms of post-traumatic stress disorder in families [19].

Nutrition: ICU patients are at an increased risk of catabolism and muscle loss, which contributes to ICU-acquired muscle weakness. Thus, the adequate provision of nutrition is important for the recovery and prevention of PICS. A dietitian should be involved to assess appropriate nutritional requirements, as overfeeding could be counterproductive.

ICU Environment: Patient and family-friendly changes, such as reducing noise, providing natural light, dimming overhead lights during sleep time, and allowing family members at the bedside, can help reduce delirium, which is the greatest risk factor for long-term cognitive impairment [20].

ICU follow-up clinics are designed to offer aftercare to ICU survivors after they are discharged. This concept is more widespread in Europe than in other regions. A study of intensive care follow-up clinics in the UK found that 30% of units had a post-ICU clinic. Financial constraints were cited as the reason for not having a post-ICU clinic. Most of the clinics were led by a nurse, and the majority of them use a locally derived health-screening questionnaire to evaluate a patient's functional recovery. Others use the short form survey-36 (SF-36), which measures health-related quality of life, and the hospital anxiety and depression scale (HADS).

There is no fixed format for ICU follow-up clinics and there is also no universally accepted method for evaluation and management [21].

However, the results of research studies on follow-up clinics have not shown many benefits. For example, in the *PRaCTICaL study*, a pragmatic non-blinded, multicenter, randomized controlled trial examined the usefulness of follow-up clinics. The study did not find any significant benefit of ICU follow-up clinics. Moreover, they found that these clinics were not cost-effective [22].

The study had several limitations. Additionally, it may simply suggest that follow-up clinics in their current format are ineffective.

A meta-analysis was conducted to evaluate the effect of follow-up ICU consultations. The analysis found that follow-up consultations may decrease PTSD symptoms in ICU survivors 3-6 months after discharge, but do not have an impact on quality of life or other outcomes [23].

84   Intensive Care

There are several barriers to ICU follow-up clinics. First, it is unclear who is the best person to lead the clinics given the multidisciplinary nature of PICS-related problems. ICU doctors and nurses trained in acute care are not well-versed in chronic problems faced by ICU survivors. Additionally, follow-up clinics at the hospital may not be convenient for patients who are already weak and have psychological issues, resulting in poor compliance. Home visits and home-based rehabilitation may be feasible, as the REACH study conducted in the Netherlands showed that home-based interdisciplinary rehabilitation is feasible for ICU survivors post-discharge. However, whether such programs are cost-effective and can be implemented in other countries needs to be evaluated.

ICU survivors should be evaluated by a multidisciplinary team of physiotherapists, occupational therapists, dietitians, speech therapists, clinical psychologists, and neuropsychiatrists for specific problems of PICS before discharge from the hospital so that follow-up can be tailored according to the needs of the patient. Follow-up can be ensured through regular telephonic interviews and telemedicine to ensure patient convenience.

Every country must create a follow-up mechanism for ICU survivors that suits their local environment and is in accordance with the resources available.

Some patients may be discharged with a tracheostomy tube, and they may or may not need ventilator support at home. These patients have unique needs, and their families must adjust accordingly. A tracheostomy is a surgical opening in the front of the neck that provides an alternate airway for breathing. It is performed on patients who cannot protect their airways or require long-term ventilator support. Tracheostomy also facilitates the removal of mucus and secretions from the airway. Before a patient with a tracheostomy is discharged, their family or caregiver should receive training on how to care for the tracheostomy tube, including cleaning and changing tubes, understanding the role of the tracheostomy cuff and the pressure required in the cuff, the role of the inner tracheostomy tube, using a suction catheter and suction machine to clear airway secretions, identifying tracheostomy tube blockage, and what to do in emergency situations. Patients who require ventilator support need a reliable electrical supply and a backup in case of outages. They may also require an oxygen concentrator or oxygen cylinders if they need a higher concentration of oxygen. Spare tubing, connectors, and an AMBU bag for manual ventilation in case of any ventilator malfunction should be available. A support system should be in place in case of emergencies.

Patients with tracheostomy have difficulty swallowing and speaking. They require the assistance of a speech therapist who can gradually teach them how to speak with a tracheostomy in place and help them with swallowing. However, patients who require continuous ventilator support may not be able to speak and need alternative means of communication. These patients have complex needs, and their rehabilitation requires a commitment from both healthcare professionals and family members.

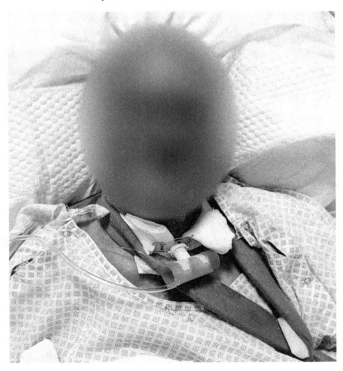

A patient with tracheostomy in place

REFERENCES:

1. A systematic review reported a 40% incidence of ICU-acquired weakness. Appleton RT, Kinsella J, Quasim T. The incidence of intensive care unit-acquired weakness syndromes: A systematic review. J Intensive Care Soc. 2015;16(2):126-136.

2. Herridge MS, Tansey CM, Matté A, et al; Canadian Critical Care Trials Group. Functional disability 5 years after acute respiratory distress syndrome. N Engl J Med. 2011; 364(14):1293-304.

3. Harvey MA, Davidson JE. Post-intensive care syndrome: right care, right now…and later. Crit Care Med 2016; 44: 381–385.

4. Pandharipande PP, Girard TD, Jackson JC, et al. Long-term cognitive impairment after critical illness. N Engl J Med 2013 369: 1306–1316.

5. Marcantonio ER, Juarez G, Goldman L, et al. The relationship of postoperative delirium with psychoactive medications. JAMA. 1994; 272(19):1518-22.

6. Myers EA, Smith DA, Allen SR, Kaplan LJ. Post-ICU syndrome: Rescuing the undiagnosed. JAAPA. 2016; 29(4):34-7.

7. Parker AM, SricharoenchaI T, Raparla S, Schneck KW, Bienvenu OJ, Needham DM. Posttraumatic stress disorder in critical illness survivors: a meta-analysis. Crit Care Med. 2015; 43(5):1121-9.

8. Harvey MA. The truth about consequences—post-intensive care syndrome in intensive care unit survivors and their families. Crit Care Med. 2012;40(8):2506-2507.

9. Davidson JE, Jones C, Bienvenu OJ: Family response to critical illness: Post intensive care syndrome-family. Crit Care Med 2012; 40:618–624

10. Jezierska N: Psychological reactions in family members of patients hospitalized in intensive care units. Anaesthesiol Intensive Ther 2014; 46:42–45.

11. Hopkins RO, Girard TD. Medical and economic implications of cognitive and psychiatric disability of survivorship. Semin Respir Crit Care Med. 2012;33(4):348-356.

12. Needham DM, Davidson J, Cohen H, et al: Improving long-term outcomes after discharge from intensive care unit: Report from a stakeholders' conference. Crit Care Med 2012; 40:502–509.

13. Elliott D, Davidson JE, Harvey MA, et al: Exploring the scope of post intensive care syndrome therapy and care: Engagement of non-critical care providers and survivors in a second stakeholders meeting. Crit Care Med 2014; 42:2518–2526.

14. Thrive. Available at: http://www.sccm.org/research/quality/thrive/Pages/default.aspx. Accessed December 11, 2015.

15. Castro E, Turcinovic M, Platz J, et al: Early mobilization: Changing the mindset. Crit Care Nurse 2015; 35:e1–e6.

16. Fuke R, HifumI T, Kondo Y et al. Early rehabilitation to prevent post intensive care syndrome in patients with critical illness: a systematic review and meta-analysis. BMJ Open 2018; 8: e019998.

17. Parker A, SricharoenchaI T, Needham DM: Early rehabilitation in the intensive care unit: Preventing physical and mental health impairments. Curr Phys Med Rehabil Rep 2013; 1:307–314.

18. Garrouste-Orgeas M, Coquet I, Perier A et al. Impact of an intensive care unit diary on psychological distress in patients and relatives*. Crit. Care Med. 2012; 40: 2033–40.

19. Jones C, Bäckman C, Griffiths RD: Intensive care diaries and relatives' symptoms of posttraumatic stress disorder after critical illness: A pilot study. Am J Crit Care 2012; 21:172–176.

20. Litton E, Carnegie V, Elliott R, Webb SA. The efficacy of earplugs as a sleep hygiene strategy for reducing delirium in the ICU: a systematic review and meta-analysis. Crit. Care Med. 2016; 44: 992–9.

21. Griffiths JA, Barber VS, Cuthbertson BH, Young JD. A national survey of intensive care follow-up clinics. Anaesthesia. 2006; 61(10):950-5.

22. Cuthbertson BH, Rattray J, Campbell MK,et al; PRaCTICaL study group. The PRaCTICaL study of nurse-led, intensive care follow-up programmes for improving long term outcomes from critical illness: a pragmatic randomised controlled trial. BMJ. 2009; 339:b3723.

23. Jensen JF, Thomsen T, Overgaard D, Bestle MH, Christensen D, Egerod I. Impact of follow-up consultations for ICU survivors on post-ICU syndrome: a systematic review and meta-analysis. Intensive Care Med. 2015; 41(5):763-75.

CHAPTER 12

BURNOUT AMONG ICU STAFF

Dr. Yogesh Manhas

Saving the lives of critically ill patients provides a sense of accomplishment and fulfillment, but working in the ICU can be stressful. High and unpredictable workloads, high patient mortality, the need for quick decision-making, distraught families demanding answers, and difficult ethical situations take a toll on the mental and physical health of ICU healthcare professionals. Burnout Syndrome is a psychological condition experienced at the workplace, characterized by emotional exhaustion, depersonalization, and a feeling of lack of personal accomplishment. Staff working in the ICU are particularly at high risk of burnout syndrome, with studies reporting up to 70% of burnout in ICU nurses and doctors [1-3]. The recent COVID-19 pandemic saw increased burnout among ICU nurses, with one study reporting 37.5% experiencing anxiety symptoms, 29.5% experiencing depressive symptoms, 78.5% feeling stressed out, and 65.5% reporting burnout [4].

Burnout was initially defined by Herbert J. Freudenberger in 1974 [5]. It typically appears approximately one year after an individual starts working in an organization. Physical symptoms include exhaustion, fatigue, frequent headaches, gastrointestinal issues, insomnia, and shortness of breath. There are also behavioral changes such as anger, frustration, irritation, paranoia, and occasionally, risk-taking behavior. In 2001, Maslach et al created a validated tool, the Maslach Burnout Inventory (MBI), to assess burnout syndrome [6].

Several factors have been identified that may trigger stress and burnout among ICU healthcare professionals.

i. Age :
Young age is a risk factor for burnout. This may be because of the lack of experience and self-confidence that comes with youth. A study found that burnout was more prevalent in individuals under the age of 40 [7].
Another study found that increased age was associated with high resilience among ICU nurses [8].

ii. Gender:
Female intensivists are at an increased risk of burnout [9].
Interestingly, a Swiss multicentre study found that a high proportion of females in the ICU nursing team was associated with decreased burnout [10].

iii. Marital Status:
Studies have reported a higher incidence of burnout among individuals who are single and do not have children [11,12].

iv. Work experience:
Several studies have found an association between less experience of working in the ICU and high rates of burnout. Perhaps those with less experience may find it difficult to handle the high and complex workload of the ICU, and are unable to prioritize their work [13,14].

v. Organizational factors:
High workload, inability to choose days off, night shifts, and rapid patient turnover are associated with increased burnout. On-call duties for more than 36 hours per week are associated with an increased risk of burnout [15,16].

vi. Ethical issues:
There is an increased prevalence of burnout among ICU doctors and nurses who deal with end-of-life decisions like withholding and withdrawal of care [17].

vii. Personality :
Neuroticism is linked to a heightened risk of burnout. It is a personality trait that is connected to negative emotions, weak

self-control, intense response to perceived threats, and a tendency to complain. Conversely, extroverted and agreeable personalities are less susceptible to burnout [18].

viii. Work relationship:
Interpersonal conflicts between nurses and physicians, peers and colleagues, supervisors, and patients and families are linked to a higher risk of burnout. A positive and high-quality relationship with the team can prevent burnout.

ix. Remuneration:
Poor salaries and compensation are a major stressor among employees in various sectors, including healthcare. Intensive care is a highly stressful job, and healthcare professionals working in the ICU deserve salaries that justify their hard work. Low salaries are the top factor driving workplace stress, according to the American Psychological Association's 2021 Work and Well-being survey. Studies have also reported inadequate salaries as the reason for burnout among nursing staff [19].

Burnout not only affects an individual but impacts the whole organization adversely. It can cause severe depression, anxiety, and post-traumatic stress disorder and unfortunately, at times healthcare staff has taken extreme steps [20]. Furthermore, there are associations between levels of burnout and staff absenteeism, low job satisfaction, poor organizational commitment, and also coronary heart disease [21].

Burnout among staff affects the quality of care and patient satisfaction. A study reported that major medical errors were linked to burnout among American surgeons [22,23].

Another study found a significant association between nurse burnout and increased urinary tract infections and surgical site infections in the hospital [24].

A staff who is under severe stress cannot exhibit empathy, thus it may lead to the dehumanization of the patients who are under his/her care. In addition, burnout results in greater sickness leaves, absenteeism, and high staff attrition rates. This causes a significant healthcare burden. Hiring new staff is not only expensive but also new staff may not be experienced and take a while to adjust to a new system. The average cost to replace an ICU nurse in the United States ranges from \$36,657 to \$88,000, causing a significant economic impact on healthcare systems [25].

Several organizations have recognized the severe negative impact of burnout on both individuals and healthcare systems, and have called for a comprehensive strategy to address it. In 2016, the Critical Care Societies Collaborative, which comprises the American Thoracic Society, the American Association of Critical Care Nurses, the American College of Chest Physicians, and the Society of Critical Care Medicine, established a working group to concentrate on the psychological health and well-being of critical care providers. The National Academy of Medicine has developed a plan to evaluate and enhance the well-being of healthcare professionals [26].

WHAT CAN BE DONE TO REDUCE BURNOUT?

Interventions are needed at both the organizational and individual levels to mitigate the risk of burnout. Burnout can be described as a bad relationship between an individual and their workplace. The six categories of person-job mismatch are...

Workload, control, reward, community, fairness and values.

These mismatches are described after several surveys and interviews of more than 10,000 people across a wide range of organizations in different countries. The six-category framework is used to assess and manage burnout [27].

i. Workload:
The high and unpredictable workload of the ICU is a risk factor. Providing adequate manpower so that every staff member has reasonable work hours to balance his/her personal and professional life is an important intervention to reduce burnout.

At an individual level, seek the help of each other and distribute work so that no single staff is overworked.

ii. Reward:
As discussed earlier, inadequate salaries are among the top stressors in the workplace. Salaries should justify the work done by ICU staff and be commensurate with the high workload, shift duties, acuity with which staff needs to attend to patients, and stress of challenging ethical issues. Unfortunately, at many healthcare organizations, ICU staff is not well compensated compared to their peers.

iii. Community:
Having good relations among colleagues is protective against burnout. Creating a support system among team members to help each other in need reduces work stress. Team debriefings after high-stress team events like cardiac arrest help improve interpersonal communication. Acknowledging and applauding the team's valuable efforts keeps morale high. During rounds, the team leader must encourage and invite suggestions from team members regarding patient management. Moreover, team-building and communication training through professional development activities can improve working relationships and conflict management.

iv. Fairness:
Favoritism at the workplace is ugly and creates a toxic environment. Everyone must have an equal opportunity. There should be a well-established and transparent mechanism for promotions.

v. Values:
Core values are beliefs that a person prioritizes the most. It can be upsetting and detrimental to work in an organization that has a value system that clashes with one's own. For instance, if someone values providing quality care to patients but works in a setting where care is subpar due to organizational reasons, they may eventually experience burnout. Likewise, a person who values family may feel stressed because they are unable to spend quality time with their family due to long work hours.

vi. Control:
Micromanagement is a pattern of manager behavior that is characterized by excessive supervision and control of employees' work and processes, as well as limited delegation of tasks or decisions to staff. Studies and surveys have demonstrated that micromanagement reduces staff productivity and efficiency [28].

Micromanagement of trained and experienced staff is a futile endeavor and counterproductive. Let staff members be accountable to each other. Furthermore, staff should have the freedom to manage their roster, leaves, and quality improvement activities. More autonomy for staff reduces stress and improves their performance.

Accountability without privilege is a source of frustration in the workplace. Consider a scenario where an ICU in-charge identifies low nurse-to-patient ratio and overcrowding as causes of a high infection rate. However, the hospital authorities hold the power to address the issue, and state approval and funding are necessary. The mismatch between accountability and the privilege to act contributes to stress and burnout.

Individuals also have a responsibility to adopt a healthy lifestyle that helps in becoming more resilient, like avoiding excess alcohol, exercising, getting adequate sleep, and engaging and fostering relationships with colleagues.

Burnout syndrome among ICU staff is damaging to the specialty of intensive care medicine. It could prevent medical and nursing students from choosing intensive care medicine as a career option. Additionally, burnout significantly affects the quality of care and triggers the dehumanization of patients.

REFERENCES:

1. Embriaco N, Azoulay E, Barrau K, Kentish N, Pochard F, Loundou A, Papazian L. High level of burnout in intensivists: prevalence and associated factors. Am J Respir Crit Care Med 2007;175: 686–692.
2. van Mol MM, Kompanje EJ, Benoit DD, Bakker J, Nijkamp MD. The Prevalence of Compassion Fatigue and Burnout among Healthcare

Professionals in Intensive Care Units: A Systematic Review. PLoS One. 2015;10(8):e0136955.

3. Costa DK, Moss M. The Cost of Caring: Emotion, Burnout, and Psychological Distress in Critical Care Clinicians. Ann Am Thorac Soc. 2018;15(7):787-790.

4. Melnyk BM, Tan A, Hsieh AP, et al. Critical care nurses' physical and mental health, worksite wellness support, and medical errors. Am J Crit Care. 2021;30(3):176-184.

5. Freudenberger, H.J. Staff burn-out. J. Soc. Issues 1974, 30, 159–165.

6. Maslach, C.; Schaufeli, W.; Leiter, M. Job burnout. Annu. Rev. Psychol. 2001, 52, 397–422.

7. MerlanI P, Verdon M, Businger A, et al. Burnout in ICU caregivers: a multicenter study of factors associated to centers. Am J Respir Crit Care Med 2011;184:1140–6.

8. Mealer M, Jones J, Newman J, et al. The presence of resilience is associated with a healthier psychological profile in intensive care unit (ICU) nurses: results of a national survey. Int J Nurs Stud 2012;49:292–9.

9. Embriaco N, Azoulay E, Barrau K, Kentish N, Pochard F, Loundou A, Papazian L. High level of burnout in intensivists: prevalence and associated factors. Am J Respir Crit Care Med. 2007;175(7):686-92.

10. MerlanI P, Verdon M, Businger A, DomenighettI G, Pargger H, Ricou B; STRESI+ Group. Burnout in ICU caregivers: a multicenter study of factors associated to centers. Am J Respir Crit Care Med. 2011;184(10):1140-6.

11. Ayala E, Carnero AM. Determinants of burnout in acute and critical care military nursing personnel: a cross-sectional study from Peru. PLoS One. 2013;8(1):e54408.

12. Chen SM, McMurray A. "Burnout" in intensive care nurses. J Nurs Res. 2001;9(5):152-64.

13. Filho, F.; Rodrigues, M.; Cimiotti, J. Burnout in Brazilian Intensive Care Units: A Comparison of Nurses and Nurse Technicians. AACN Adv. Crit. Care 2019, 30, 16–21.

14. Aytekin A, Yilmaz F, Kuguoglu S. Burnout levels in neonatal intensive care nurses and its effects on their quality of life. Aust J Adv Nurs2013;31:39–47.

15. Cañadas-De la Fuente, G.A.; Albendín-García, L.; de la Fuente, E.; San Luis, C.; Gómez-Urquiza, J.L.; Cañadas, G. Burnout in Nursing Professionals Performing Overtime Workdays in Emergency and Critical Care Departments. Rev. Esp. Salud. Publica 2016, 90, e1-9.

16. Poncet MC, Toullic P, Papazian L, et al. Burnout syndrome in critical care nursing staff. Am J Respir Crit Care Med. 2007;175:698–704.

17. Teixeira C, Ribeiro O, Fonseca AM, et al. Burnout in intensive care units -a consideration of the possible prevalence and frequency of new risk factors: A descriptive co-relational multicentre study. BMC Anesthesiol2013;13:38.

18. Myhren H, Ekeberg Ø, Stokland O. Job satisfaction and burnout among intensive care unit nurses and physicians. Crit Care Res Pract2013;2013:6.

19. SarabI RE, Javanmard R, ShahrbabakI PM. Study of burnout syndrome, job satisfaction, and related factors among health care workers in rural areas of Southeastern Iran. AIMS Public Health. 2020;7(1):158-168.

20. Awan S, Diwan MN, Aamir A, Allahuddin Z, Irfan M, Carano A, Vellante F, Ventriglio A, Fornaro M, Valchera A, Pettorruso M, MartinottI G, DI Giannantonio M, Ullah I, De Berardis D. Suicide in Healthcare Workers: Determinants, Challenges, and the Impact of COVID-19. Front Psychiatry. 2022;12:792925.

21. Reader TW, Cuthbertson BH, Decruyenaere J. Burnout in the ICU: potential consequences for staff and patient well-being. Intensive Care Med. 2008;34(1):4-6.

22. Shanafelt TD, Balch CM, Bechamps G, Russell T, Dyrbye L, Satele D, Collicott P, Novotny PJ, Sloan J, Freischlag J. Burnout and medical errors among American surgeons. Ann Surg. 2010;251(6):995-1000.

23. Vahey DC, Aiken LH, Sloane DM, Clarke SP, Vargas D. Nurse burnout and patient satisfaction. Med Care. 2004;42(2 Suppl):II57-66.

24. CimiottI JP, Aiken LH, Sloane DM, Wu ES. Nurse staffing, burnout, and health care-associated infection. Am J Infect Control. 2012;40(6):486-90.

25. Kurnat-Thoma E, Ganger M, Peterson K, Channell L. Reducing annual hospital and registered nurse staff turnover—a 10 element on boarding program intervention. SAGE Open Nurs. 2017;3:1–13.

26. National Academy of Medicine Action Collaborative on Clinician Well-Being and Resilience. Validated Instruments to Assess Work-Related Dimensions of Well-Being.

27. Maslach, C., & Leiter, M. P. (2005). Reversing Burnout. Stanford Social Innovation Review, 3(4), 43–49.

28. DeCaro MS, Thomas RD, Albert NB, Beilock SL. Choking under pressure: multiple routes to skill failure. J Exp Psychol Gen. 2011;140(3):390-406.

CHAPTER 13

MAKING SENSE OF RANDOMIZED CONTROLLED TRIALS IN INTENSIVE CARE

Dr. Abhijit Nair, Dr. Yogesh Manhas

Randomized controlled trials (RCTs) are considered the gold standard for evaluating the efficacy of interventions in healthcare [1]. Conducting a well-designed, appropriately powered RCT not only requires an adequate number of like-minded researchers and a research environment, but also proper training, a lot of time, and patience. One must not forget the cost incurred for such studies, which are impossible without the support of the organization. There are a lot of logistics involved, such as ethical clearance, trial registration, randomization, follow-ups, data collection and analysis, and finally, manuscript writing [2].

Conducting randomized controlled trials (RCTs) in critically ill patients admitted to the intensive care unit (ICU) can be challenging. The ICU environment has unique features, such as the severity of illness, rapid changes in clinical status, and the use of complex therapeutic interventions, which can affect the design, implementation, and interpretation of RCTs in this setting [3]. One of the main concerns in conducting RCTs in critically ill patients is the issue of informed consent. Many critically ill patients are unable to provide informed consent due to their medical condition, and surrogate decision-makers may not be available or may not have sufficient information to make informed decisions. This can lead to ethical and legal issues, as well as challenges in obtaining regulatory approval for the study [4].

Another concern is the potential for confounding and bias. Confounding occurs when an intervention has an effect that is independent of the treatment being studied, and this can compromise the validity of the trial results. In the ICU, multiple interventions are often given simultaneously, making it difficult to determine the true effect of a single intervention. Bias can occur when patients or healthcare providers are aware of the study treatment, leading to a difference in the care received or reported outcomes between the study groups. In a study by Dahlberg et al, the authors analyzed the barriers and challenges in the process of including critically ill patients in an RCT [5]. The authors concluded that the inclusion process led to the omission of nearly three out of four eligible patients. In their study, the obstacles in the recruitment process were practical, medical, legal, or ethical. The majority of critically sick patients in the ICU were unable to provide written, informed consent for inclusion. The authors discovered that the issue of preserving autonomy and competence to consent was difficult among patients who gave consent. Even when patients seemed to be competent, some were unable to recollect what they had consented to, and others appeared unable to distinguish between research and treatment. The employment of next of kin as surrogate decision-makers adds further concerns.

Additionally, the high risk of adverse events and death in critically ill patients can limit the feasibility and acceptability of RCTs. The use of invasive or experimental interventions in critically ill patients may increase the risk of harm, which can make it difficult to obtain ethical approval for the study. Moreover, the high mortality rate in the ICU can make it difficult to enroll sufficient numbers of patients or to complete the study, potentially leading to Type II errors or insufficient power to detect significant differences between the study groups [6-8].

Another concern is the rapid changes in clinical status that can occur in critically ill patients. This can result in unexpected withdrawals from the study, incomplete data collection, or changes in the primary endpoint of the study, making it difficult to interpret the results. Additionally, the use of life-support interventions, such as mechanical ventilation, can affect the ability to assess outcomes, such as patient-centered outcomes or quality of life, leading to challenges in the interpretation of the results.

98   Intensive Care

Furthermore, the use of standard-of-care interventions, such as antimicrobial therapy, can vary widely between ICUs, making it difficult to generalize the results of RCTs to other ICUs. The use of multiple co-interventions and the complexity of care in the ICU can also make it challenging to determine the true effect of the intervention being studied.

The pendulum effect occurs when a study shows a positive or beneficial effect of an intervention, but is later followed by a study that shows no effect or even a negative effect. This can be stressful and confusing for Intensivists. An example of the pendulum effect is the use of hydroxy-chloroquine in COVID-19 pneumonia patients during the pandemic [9].

According to Niven et al, the most effective approach to closing the quality gap will be through quality improvement and education. This will also establish the foundation for future practical RCTs that will provide the necessary solutions for both our practice and our patients [10].

In 2019, Hernandez et al published the results of the ANDROMEDA-SHOCK trial in a paper titled 'Effect of a Resuscitation Strategy Targeting Peripheral Perfusion Status versus Serum Lactate Levels on 28-Day Mortality Among Patients With Septic Shock: The ANDROMEDA-SHOCK Randomized Clinical Trial' in the reputable journal JAMA [11]. The objective of this study was to determine if peripheral perfusion–targeted resuscitation during early septic shock in adults is more effective than a lactate level–targeted resuscitation for reducing mortality. The study enrolled 416 critically-ill patients into 2 groups: in one group, the aim was to normalize the capillary refilling time, and in the other group, the aim was to reduce serum lactate levels. The authors concluded that a resuscitation strategy targeting normalization of capillary refill time, compared with a strategy targeting serum lactate levels, did not reduce all-cause 28-day mortality in septic shock. The researchers used frequentist statistical methods for data analysis in this paper.

In 2020, ZampierI et al reevaluated the findings of the ANDROMEDA-SHOCK trial using Bayesian and frequentist methods [12]. They determined that resuscitation targeted at peripheral perfusion may lead to reduced mortality and quicker resolution of organ dysfunction compared to a lactate-targeted strategy. However, the conflicting results from the same data using different methods can be perplexing for intensivists and do not offer clear guidance on which approach is superior.

Finally, the logistics of conducting RCTs in the ICU can be challenging. The need for close monitoring and frequent reassessment of the patient can limit the ability to conduct trials in a blinded manner, potentially compromising the validity of the results. The availability of staff and resources, such as personnel to obtain informed consent or perform the intervention, can also be limited in the ICU.

The majority of study trials in intensive care medicine focus on reducing mortality and use it as an endpoint. However, the relevance of mortality as an endpoint is questionable due to the complex and heterogeneous condition of ICU patients, which is affected by numerous confounding factors such as medicine, equipment, human, and organizational factors. It is difficult to control all these factors. Moreover, the outcome of critically ill patients depends on a bundle of interventions with positive effects rather than a single intervention. In a systematic review of 72 randomized controlled trials in intensive care, only ten trials showed a reduction in mortality, while 55 trials reported no effect on mortality [13]. Additionally, the positive results of many trials were not replicated in subsequent larger trials Choosing mortality as the endpoint can negate the immediate positive effect of the studied intervention, giving readers the impression that the intervention was not useful. For instance, a study comparing two fluid management strategies in acute lung injury did not find any mortality benefit, but the group with conservative fluid strategy showed improved oxygenation [14].

Similarly, initial trials with prone positioning in acute respiratory distress syndrome did not show any reduction in mortality but did improve the oxygenation of the patients [15]. The prone position was not commonly used in acute respiratory distress syndrome until the PROSEVA trial published in 2013 demonstrated a decrease in mortality

100   Intensive Care

[16]. We should consider whether relying too heavily on mortality reduction delays the adoption of an otherwise beneficial intervention.

There are examples where the use of mortality as an endpoint to find a difference seems irrelevant. For example, comparing two sedation strategies using mortality as an endpoint seems to be an oversimplification of a complex situation of critically ill patients from diverse etiologies.

There are also concerns when the standard practice of care is altered in the control group during the design of randomized control trials. The Acute Respiratory Distress Syndrome (ARDS) Network trial of low tidal volume ventilation used higher tidal volumes of 10-12ml/ kg predicted body weight in the control group, which some experts argue was not the standard practice at that time [17].

Another problem with randomized controlled trials in the ICU is the concept of *practice misalignment*. The condition of critically ill patients is very dynamic, and thus therapies need to be titrated, be it fluids, vasopressors, blood transfusions, or ventilator settings. But for the sake of practicality and feasibility, patients are often randomized into two fixed therapy protocols, ignoring the changing severity of the disease in the randomized patients. Such an approach may result in some randomized patients receiving excessive therapy while others receive less than the required therapy. This gives rise to *practice misalignment*. The Canadian Transfusion Requirements in Critical Care (TRICC) Trial randomized adequately resuscitated critically ill patients who were not actively bleeding to one of two fixed hemoglobin transfusion triggers, a liberal (10 g/dL hemoglobin) or restrictive (7 g/dL) threshold, independent of comorbidities. The results of the study found that the hospital mortality rate was significantly higher in the liberal strategy group compared with the restrictive strategy group. Based on these findings, the authors concluded that most critically ill patients should only receive red cell transfusions when their hemoglobin concentration is 7.0 g/dL [18].

However, when investigating transfusion practices prior to the study's randomization, it was discovered that the blood transfusion threshold was influenced by various factors such as age, illness severity, the existence of ischemic heart disease, anemia, and shock. Therefore, blood transfusion was adjusted according to several patient factors before the study, but this was not considered during the study [19].

Perhaps experts in intensive care medicine need to rethink how the trials should be conducted and what the appropriate endpoints are to get meaningful answers [20].

Improving clinically meaningful and patient-centered outcomes should be the core of research in the ICU. The research should concentrate on interventions that may improve quality of life, lower the cost of treatment, and can be easily implemented if the results are positive and encouraging [21].

ALTERNATIVE TO RCTS FOR RESEARCH IN ICU:

Observational studies:

Observational studies, compared to RCTs, are typically quick, inexpensive, and easy to carry out. They can be much larger than RCTs, making it possible to investigate a rare outcome. When an RCT would be unethical, an observational study can be used instead. However, unlike clinical trials, observational research cannot control for bias and confounding [22].

The prerequisites for a well-designed observational study are a detailed patient's exposure history, past medical history, co-morbidities, medications, time-varying events, and risk measures during the illness. Furthermore, to reduce systematic error, the design of research seeking observational inference involves previous information—often from subject matter experts regarding predictors of exposure and outcome as well as statistical approaches for dealing with random error [23].

Adaptive trials can answer research questions more efficiently and effectively than traditional RCTs, but they require extensive and far more complex statistical preparation. An adaptive design allows

102 Intensive Care

modifications to the trial and/or statistical procedures of the trial after its initiation without undermining its validity and integrity. The purpose is to make clinical trials more flexible, efficient, and fast. The adoption of adaptive trials on a larger scale is projected to enhance the cost-benefit ratio of clinical studies in critically ill patients [24].

When compared to RCTs, adaptive designs may offer several advantages. Patients have a higher chance of receiving better therapy. Researchers and funders may be able to answer research questions with fewer patients, resulting in a more efficient use of research resources.

The complexities of adaptive trial statistical analysis should not be underestimated. First, the numerous intermediate analyses require accounting for repeated testing. Second, imbalanced baseline characteristics may occur within subgroups due to low numbers, which must be accounted for at each interim analysis.

Thirdly, time trends may confound effects if response adaptive randomization is used. Fourth, normal methods cannot calculate operational features such as predicted sample size and the likelihood of inaccurate findings as more adaptations are adopted, and simulation studies must determine them. Therefore, trained statisticians must be involved, and a complete statistical analysis plan detailing all possible adjustments must be prepared before the study begins.

In conclusion, conducting RCTs in critically ill patients admitted to the ICU can be challenging due to the unique features of the ICU environment, including the severity of illness, rapid changes in clinical status, and the use of complex therapeutic interventions [25].

The need for informed consent, the potential for confounding and bias, the high risk of adverse events and death, rapid changes in clinical status, the use of standard-of-care interventions, and the logistics of conducting trials can all impact the design, implementation, and interpretation of RCTs in this setting. Despite these challenges, RCTs in critically ill patients are important for advancing our understanding of the best treatments and improving the quality of care for this vulnerable population.

REFERENCES:

1. Hariton E, Locascio JJ. Randomised controlled trials - the gold standard for effectiveness research: Study design: randomised controlled trials. BJOG. 2018; 125(13):1716.

2. Djurisic S, Rath A, Gaber S, et al. Barriers to the conduct of randomised clinical trials within all disease areas. Trials. 2017; 18(1):3601. Hariton E, Locascio JJ. Randomised controlled trials - the gold standard for effectiveness research: Study design: randomised controlled trials. BJOG. 2018; 125(13):1716.

3. Djurisic S, Rath A, Gaber S, et al. Barriers to the conduct of randomised clinical trials within all disease areas. Trials. 2017; 18(1):360.

4. Hébert PC, Cook DJ, Wells G, Marshall J. The design of randomized clinical trials in critically ill patients. Chest. 2002; 121(4):1290-300.

5. Luce JM. Is the concept of informed consent applicable to clinical research involving critically ill patients? Crit Care Med. 2003; 31(3 Suppl):S153-60.

6. Dahlberg J, Eriksen C, Robertsen A, Beitland S. Barriers and challenges in the process of including critically ill patients in clinical studies. Scand J Trauma ResuscEmerg Med. 2020; 28(1):51.

7. Vincent JL. We should abandon randomized controlled trials in the intensive care unit. Crit Care Med. 2010 Oct;38(10 Suppl):S534-8.

8. Ospina-Tascón GA, Büchele GL, Vincent JL. Multicenter, randomized, controlled trials evaluating mortality in intensive care: doomed to fail? Crit Care Med. 2008; 36(4):1311-22.

9. Harhay MO, Wagner J, Ratcliffe SJ, Bet al. Outcomes and statistical power in adult critical care randomized trials. Am J Respir Crit Care Med. 2014;189(12):1469-78.

10. SattuI SE, Liew JW, Graef ER, et al. Swinging the pendulum: lessons learned from public discourse concerning hydroxychloroquine and COVID-19. Expert Rev Clin Immunol. 2020; 16(7):659-66.

11. Niven AS, Herasevich S, Pickering BW, Gajic O. The Future of Critical Care Lies in Quality Improvement and Education. Ann Am Thorac Soc. 2019;16(6): 649-656.

12. Hernández G, Ospina-Tascón GA, DamianI LP, et al. Effect of a Resuscitation Strategy Targeting Peripheral Perfusion Status vs Serum Lactate Levels on 28-Day Mortality Among Patients With Septic Shock: The ANDROMEDA-SHOCK Randomized Clinical Trial. JAMA. 2019;321(7):654-664.

13. ZampierI FG, DamianI LP, Bakker J, et al. Effects of a Resuscitation Strategy Targeting Peripheral Perfusion Status versus Serum Lactate Levels among Patients with Septic Shock. A Bayesian Reanalysis

of the ANDROMEDA-SHOCK Trial. Am J Respir Crit Care Med. 2020;201(4):423-429.

14. Ospina-Tascón GA, Büchele GL, Vincent JL. Multicenter, randomized, controlled trials evaluating mortality in intensive care: doomed to fail? Crit Care Med. 2008 Apr;36(4):1311-22.

15. National Heart, Lung, and Blood Institute Acute Respiratory Distress Syndrome (ARDS) Clinical Trials Network; Wiedemann HP, Wheeler AP, Bernard GR, et al. Comparison of two fluid-management strategies in acute lung injury. N Engl J Med. 2006 Jun 15;354(24):2564-75.

16. GattinonI L, TognonI G, PesentI A, et al; Prone-Supine Study Group. Effect of prone positioning on the survival of patients with acute respiratory failure. N Engl J Med. 2001 Aug 23;345(8):568-73.

17. Guérin C, Reignier J, Richard JC, et al; PROSEVA Study Group. Prone positioning in severe acute respiratory distress syndrome. N Engl J Med. 2013 Jun 6;368(23):2159-68.

18. Eichacker PQ, Gerstenberger EP, Banks SM, CuI X, Natanson C. Meta-analysis of acute lung injury and acute respiratory distress syndrome trials testing low tidal volumes. Am J Respir Crit Care Med. 2002;166(11):1510-4.

19. Hebert PC, Wells G, Blajchman MA, et al: A multicenter, randomized, controlled clinical trial of transfusion requirements in critical care. Transfusion Requirements in Critical Care Investigators, Canadian Critical Care Trials Group. N Engl J Med 1999; 340: 409–417.

20. Deans KJ, MinnecI PC, SuffredinI AF, et al. Randomization in clinical trials of titrated therapies: unintended consequences of using fixed treatment protocols. Crit Care Med. 2007;35(6):1509-16.

21. Vincent JL. We should abandon randomized controlled trials in the intensive care unit. Crit Care Med. 2010 Oct;38(10 Suppl):S534-8.

22. Emanuel EJ. The future of biomedical research. JAMA. 2013;309(15):1589-90.

23. Gilmartin-Thomas JF, Liew D, Hopper I. Observational studies and their utility for practice. Aust Prescr. 2018; 41(3):82-85.

24. Walkey AJ, Sheldrick RC, Kashyap R, et al. Guiding Principles for the Conduct of Observational Critical Care Research for Coronavirus Disease 2019 Pandemics and Beyond: The Society of Critical Care Medicine Discovery Viral Infection and Respiratory Illness Universal Study Registry. Crit Care Med. 2020; 48(11):e1038-e1044.

25. van Werkhoven CH, Harbarth S, Bonten MJM. Adaptive designs in clinical trials in critically ill patients: principles, advantages, and pitfalls. Intensive Care Med. 2019; 45(5):678-682.

26. Granholm A, AlhazzanI W, Derde LPG, et al. Randomised clinical trials in critical care: past, present and future. Intensive Care Med. 2022; 48(2):164-178.

CHAPTER

14   ANECDOTES

A patient in his early fifties was admitted with severe shortness of breath. A trial of noninvasive ventilation (NIV) was offered, but the patient did not show much response. His oxygen levels kept dropping despite receiving 100% oxygen. A prompt decision was taken to intubate and ventilate him. He was sedated, paralyzed, and kept on mechanical ventilation. His chest x-ray revealed bilateral infiltrates consistent with acute respiratory distress syndrome (ARDS). The patient was kept in the prone position daily as per protocols. His stay was complicated by bilateral pneumothoraces for which he required insertion of chest tubes. He had a brief cardiac arrest during the insertion of chest tubes but was revived with expeditious CPR (cardiopulmonary resuscitation). Investigations revealed H1N1 viral pneumonia. Over the next few days, he did show some improvement in his respiratory parameters, but attempts to wean him from the ventilator failed. It was clear that he would take a long time to recover, and weaning from the ventilator would not be easy, so a decision was taken to do a tracheostomy on him to facilitate weaning. However, a few days after the tracheostomy, he developed a fever and new infiltrates on X-ray suggestive of ventilator associated pneumonia. Endotracheal samples revealed Acinetobacter infection for which appropriate antibiotics were started. Over the next few days, he did show improvement on chest X-ray, but the fever did not subside. The blood samples sent for cultures reported a fungus in his blood. Without delay, antifungal was started, and an echocardiogram was also requested to rule out any fungal vegetations in the heart. Fortunately, he did respond to the treatment. He spent one and a

106 Intensive Care

half months in the ICU. Due to a long stay in the ICU with severe illness, he developed critical illness myopathy, but gradually, with the help of physiotherapy and respiratory therapy, he was taken off the ventilator and moved to the ward. A few days later, his tracheostomy tube was removed, and he was discharged home. There was no formal follow-up, but we got information that he joined back his office.

Intensive care does save lives, but it takes a tremendous amount of effort and patience from not only ICU doctors and nurses but also every department of the hospital. Coordinated care between various specialties can result in better outcomes for critically ill patients.

A 91-year-old man was admitted following a road traffic accident in which the driver lost control and the car rolled over at high speed. One of the passengers died on the spot. The patient had severe chest injuries with multiple rib fractures on both sides of the chest, underlying severe lung contusions, and blood in the pleural cavity. He also had multiple fractures of the sternum, scapula, and bones of the forearm. He was conscious on arrival and, after initial assessment, investigations, and stabilization, he was shifted to the high dependency unit for pain management. However, after a few hours, the ICU received a call that the patient became unresponsive and was having labored breathing. The ICU team, after a quick assessment, intubated and connected him to a mechanical ventilator. Blood gas revealed high carbon dioxide in the blood. Due to severe chest injuries, he was not able to breathe adequately. The patient was put on a continuous infusion of strong analgesics for pain control. After a few days, weaning from mechanical ventilation was attempted but failed. Since he was unable to make adequate cough efforts, the team realized that it would be best to perform a tracheostomy in order to facilitate weaning from the ventilator and also for tracheal toilet. After the tracheostomy, the patient was gradually weaned from ventilator support. Physiotherapists, dietitians, and respiratory therapists were active in patient rehabilitation. The patient did well and eventually, the tracheostomy tube was removed before discharge from the hospital.

Old age is not a criterion for denial of intensive care if there is a good chance of recovery.

A 58-year-old man suffered severe chest trauma after a road traffic accident. He was intubated and put on a mechanical ventilator upon arrival at Accident and Emergency as he was unconscious. He had fractures of several ribs and sternum. CT scans also revealed undisplaced fractures of multiple cervical vertebrae. There was no evidence of head injury on the CT scan. The next day, the ICU team stopped sedation to assess his neurological status. He was conscious and responsive. The team noticed that he was moving his upper limbs on command but was not able to move his lower limbs. This made the team suspicious about an injury to the spinal cord. Reflex response in lower limbs were decreased. The hospital did not have the services of an MRI or spinal surgeons, so a tertiary hospital was contacted for transfer to investigate further and provide definitive management. The team at the tertiary hospital accepted the patient, but the transfer was delayed for 48 hours due to the non-availability of a bed at the tertiary hospital.

This brings up the question of whether intensive care services should be regionalized and concentrated at tertiary hospitals, allowing for comprehensive care to be provided under one roof. Tertiary hospitals should create enough beds to accommodate patients from secondary hospitals in the catchment area. Critical patients in need of intensive care can be transferred to tertiary hospitals after initial stabilization. The efficiency of manpower utilization through regionalization of intensive care services has been previously discussed.

108   Intensive Care

A 60-year-old man was transferred to the ICU from the operating room after undergoing aortic valve replacement due to aortic stenosis. He had systemic lupus erythematosus (SLE) and was taking corticosteroids. It was standard procedure to monitor post-cardiac surgery patients in the ICU and wean them off the ventilator after a few hours of observation and stabilization. Three hours after admission to the ICU, the nurse stopped the sedation and began the process of weaning the patient off the ventilator since his vital signs were stable. Shortly after stopping the sedation, I received a distress call from the nurse to attend to the patient immediately. Upon arrival, I saw that the patient's chest drain chamber was completely filled with fresh blood, indicating a major bleed from the surgical site. We quickly collected 2 packs of O negative blood and notified the blood bank of the crisis. The cardiac surgeon was contacted who advised that the only way to save the patient was for one of the ICU doctors to open the chest and control the bleeding vessel since there was no in house cardiac surgeon. With the cardiac surgeon guiding us over the phone, we proceeded to cut the wire sutures of the sternum. By the time we cut all the wires, the cardiac surgeon had arrived and took over. The patient was bleeding from the aortic site, but the surgeon was able to stop it manually, and patient was rushed to the operating theater for definitive repair. The next day, the patient was safely taken off the ventilator and was stable. Due to acute hemodynamic instability and transfusion of multiple blood products, he suffered acute kidney injury but did not require hemodialysis support.

A well-coordinated team effort and the resourceful thinking of cardiac surgeon saved a life.

An 85-year-old man presented to emergency room with altered sensorium and low blood pressure. The ICU team was involved as the patient's conscious level was too low to protect his airway. After an intravenous fluid bolus, his blood pressure became normal. On examination, he was thin and frail. The family informed the medical team that he had not been able to eat for the last few days. He was known to have diabetes, hypertension, chronic kidney disease, ischemic heart disease, and had suffered a stroke ten months prior, which left him bedridden and unable to communicate or recognize his family members. Due to his poor baseline quality of life, the family was informed of his current condition and that life support would not achieve any meaningful outcome. The ICU team suggested investigating the patient for any infections, providing antibiotics, fluids, and nutrition through a nasogastric tube, but not any life support. The patient was also considered for DNR status. However, the family strongly objected and wanted everything done for him. There is no legislation in the country that allows medical professionals to take unilateral decisions to deny life support therapies, even if they are futile. Therefore, the patient was intubated and put on mechanical ventilation. His urine culture was positive for an infection, which responded well to antibiotics, but he could not be taken off the ventilator due to his poor conscious level. The family was advised to consider a tracheostomy, but they refused. The patient spent more than a month in the ICU before passing away due to a hospital-acquired lung infection. Since no DNR order was in place, the patient received CPR multiple times before being declared dead.

Lack of clear laws on DNR and withholding of life support decisions causes prolongation of the patient's suffering and also results in inefficient use of scarce resources.

An 80-year-old man was admitted to the ICU with septic shock. He was suffering from diabetes and hypertension. His blood sugars were poorly controlled, and he had not been compliant with his medications.

His blood gas analysis showed severe metabolic acidosis. He was given intravenous fluids and started on empirical antibiotics. Cultures for septic workup were sent. To maintain his blood pressure, vasopressors were started. However, his condition continued to deteriorate and he had to be put on a mechanical ventilator. Over the next 72 hours, the patient continued to deteriorate and there was no response to empirical antibiotics. His urine culture and blood culture

110   Intensive Care

grew the same organism which was sensitive to the antibiotic that he was receiving. He also developed acute kidney injury and his liver functions started deteriorating. At this juncture, family counseling was conducted and the patient's current condition and poor prognosis were explained. The family understood well and agreed to a DNR status. However, the team did not discuss withholding life support therapies and not escalating treatment further. Thus, the team continued increasing vasopressors to maintain blood pressure and kept requesting investigations unnecessarily.

The lack of clarity on end-of-life decisions and incomplete communication result in futile efforts, wasted manpower, increased risk of burnout among staff, and, of course, prolongation of the patient's suffering.

A 20-year-old girl was admitted to a private hospital with severe shortness of breath. Her chest x-ray showed bilateral infiltrates consistent with ARDS. Despite high flow oxygen, she was unable to maintain her oxygen levels and was intubated and put on a mechanical ventilator. Initially, she required high ventilator support, but in the next few days, her oxygen requirement started to decrease. However, after a week of stay in the ICU, her family started complaining about the cost of treatment since they had no insurance. They wanted the ICU team to get her off the ventilator, even though she clearly was not ready. They were informed that this would take more time and she may even need a tracheostomy if attempts at weaning failed. However, at the end of the second week, the family decided to take the patient out of the hospital against medical advice.

Intensive care is expensive and can become unaffordable when the patient is paying out of pocket. This is a case where intensive care services could not be fully utilized for the patient due to the financial burden on the family.

A woman in her mid-thirties with breast carcinoma that had spread to her lungs was admitted due to severe shortness of breath. She was undergoing palliative chemotherapy and was given non-invasive ventilation to aid her breathing. The ICU consultant discussed her poor prognosis and the futility of any life support intervention with her family. They were informed that the goal of ICU care was to make her as comfortable as possible, using medication to relieve her shortness of breath, pain, and anxiety. The family was reassured that a nursing staff would be assigned to care for her, and they agreed with the plan. The patient was started on a morphine infusion and a small dose of midazolam to reduce her anxiety. The family was allowed to be at her bedside, and she passed away peacefully in the next few hours.

Good communication skills and knowledge of palliative care is important for intensivists involved in the end of life care.